Kettlebell Training

Build Strong Body and Lose Weight With Kettlebell

(Burn Fat and Get Lean and Shredded in a Days With Total Body Kettlebell Training)

Erick Elliott

Published By **Bengion Cosalas**

Erick Elliott

All Rights Reserved

Kettlebell Training: Build Strong Body and Lose Weight With Kettlebell (Burn Fat and Get Lean and Shredded in a Days With Total Body Kettlebell Training)

ISBN 978-1-998927-72-2

No part of this guidebook shall be reproduced in any form without permission in writing from the publisher except in the case of brief quotations embodied in critical articles or reviews.

Legal & Disclaimer

The information contained in this book is not designed to replace or take the place of any form of medicine or professional medical advice. The information in this book has been provided for educational & entertainment purposes only.

The information contained in this book has been compiled from sources deemed reliable, and it is accurate to the best of the Author's knowledge; however, the Author cannot guarantee its accuracy and validity and cannot be held liable for any errors or omissions. Changes are periodically made to this book. You must consult your doctor or get professional medical advice before using any of the suggested remedies, techniques, or information in this book.

Table Of Contents

Chapter 1: Why Am I Getting Fat?

It sure is hard to preserve an active life-style and consume a healthful, balanced diet given the tempo of our present day lives, the development of generation, and the conveniences of rapid food. But if you recognise a manner to do it, it may be executed, regardless of a busy manner of lifestyles.

In this first chapter of the e-book, we're able to look at:

•Why keeping a schedule in reality aids in weight reduction;

•the number one reasons of weight benefit;

•the humans we ought to are in search of for recommendation from whilst we determine we are prepared to lose the weight.

•Along with many distinct subjects, mastering about weight loss secrets and techniques and strategies will help you discern out the manner to subsequently lose the weight and preserve it off absolutely.

The Principal Reasons for Weight Gain

i.We consume more energy every day than our our bodies require, and the greater is then stored as fat: We all understand this, so why are 63% of Americans overweight or obese? The portions we devour nowadays are large, as you can see.

We are in a excessive wonderful power balance whilst we devour extra than we burn. Essentially, we keep the greater as fat. If we had been cavemen and knew we would not consume for seven days, this might be a excellent difficulty, however for those folks who stay in western society, this isn't always the case.

ii. You do no longer get enough sleep: It can be time to take care of any sleep issues you can have in case you are weight loss plan and exercise however are despite the fact that now not dropping weight. In the Canadian

Medical Association Journal, Canadian obesity experts be aware that there can be growing evidence pointing to a connection amongst sleep and weight reduction. In fact, the take a look at located that those who stay up later devour four hundred–500 extra energy!

iii. Your metabolism: After the age of 25, we start to lose 10% of our metabolic price each ten years. If you take a look at the instructions on this e-book for kettlebell training, you can save you this from taking place. In exclusive words, at the same time as we've were given more lean muscle, our metabolic charge rises due to the fact our bodies want to assemble extra muscle to repair the muscle from the workout. We gain weight whilst we are sedentary due to the fact this does not take area.

iv. Your eating conduct are subpar: People in the West are really 30 pounds heavier than they have been one hundred years within the beyond, constant with my research for this e-book. They fed on extra fats, it's even extra thrilling! You see, ingredients immoderate in sugars, starches, and almost something made with flour are making us an overweight society. Fast Food Facts critiques that the short food enterprise on my own spent 4.2 billion greenbacks on marketing and advertising and marketing in 2009! We are fat for a cause. A meal planner has been positioned with the useful resource of manner of many human beings to be helpful in pointing them within the right course.

v. Larger factor sizes: This is common knowledge. Simply located, maximum humans consume an excessive amount of. This meal planner permit you to apprehend what a element need to look like, as became formerly mentioned.

vi.   Exercise or the shortage thereof: The western society is being destroyed with the useful resource of this. Today's children are the primary technology to have a shorter existence expectancy than their parents, in keeping with designedtomove.Org. The human frame is constructed for motion. To obtain and maintain a healthful weight, regular exercising is essential. What you devour, the way you eat, and what type of you devour are also important elements.

vii. Control your consumption. Use your hand to measure in choice to weighing or measuring as a easy rule of thumb in this case. Men want portions of protein, even as women exceptional want one. Your palm may suit indoors of a issue.

Both ladies and men must choose out a part of carbohydrates that is the size of your fist.

Protein this is the identical length as your palm ought to be ate up via way of guys. The majority of humans frequently underestimate how masses they may be ingesting because of this detail. Generally, you need to most effective devour a part of meals the scale of your fist at a time due to the reality this is furthermore the dimensions of your stomach.

When you're 80% complete, prevent consuming. This is a technique that I use ninety% of the time, and it's going to without a doubt assist you devour much less. Consider detail control in this situation; there is no higher manner to manipulate what you install your mouth than with the beneficial useful resource of ingesting a whole lot much less at each meal. If you try this for a yr, you could lose quite a few weight.

Try eating greater slowly and keep away from consuming on the same time as using, standing, or shifting. You need to handiest eat meals at a table. You need to devour slowly due to the fact your thoughts receives a signal at the same time as you're complete.

When you devour fast, your mind does not get keep of the signal, main you to overeat due to the fact you do not sense "complete." I apprehend you're busy, but in case you alternative a healthful meal for one whilst you are busy, you may although be able to hold a healthy weight.

Of route, monitoring your intake of fatty and sugary meals is some other vital step. To stay balanced, anybody want vitamins, together with healthful fats, however ingesting masses of junk meals and sugary beverages will substantially contribute to our weight benefit. Processed components are normally low in nutrients, in the occasion that they include any the least bit, and high in horrible fats, salt, and sugar.

People frequently blame their busy schedules for their weight benefit. To avoid falling into any traps a brilliant way to strain you to make horrible vitamins selections, you need to absolutely plan in advance in this situation.

You can plan your food for the week and get a shopping for list for all of the substances you could want with a meal planner.

Breakfast may be hard to healthy in, so that you can avoid creating a terrible choice or going with out meals altogether, I recommend using a meal opportunity.

Do I Need to Start A Diet?

The brief reaction is "actually not" They are not prolonged-time period solutions. It's difficult to keep away from falling for the hype at the same time because the maximum up to date "weight-reduction plan fad" is carefully marketed, as we've got already stated. Think approximately a way of life exchange in area of a weight loss program due to the truth this could create long-term healthy ingesting and exercising conduct in place of a brief restoration eating regimen.

Do you revel in skipping whole meals groups like carbohydrates or chugging down weight reduction beverages that truely do no longer flavor first-rate or fill you up?

Most human beings appear to begin a food regimen around large life activities, together with marriage, high college or family reunions, or the massive one—New Year's resolutions.

If reaching a healthful weight is your first-rate purpose, I would endorse you to do your studies. At least you'll be aware about the manner to keep the load off ultimately as soon as you've got have been given reached your quick-term goal.

You want to have a purpose for making any sort of exchange to your regular every day sports earlier than you begin. These might be appeared as objectives or dreams.

Goals are important because of the fact with out them, you'll surrender even as subjects get hard. Perhaps you recently went from a length 40 to a period forty in pants, and you're sick of being huge. Maybe your clinical health practitioner warned you that during case you do not lose 50 pounds, a coronary coronary heart assault is a real possibility.

Your goals have to be sincere. Writing them down permits you to reveal them somewhere and be reminded of them each day. The acronym S.M.A.R.T. Is the gadget I prefer to use.

Specific: Starting out with best a indistinct idea of in that you're going will guarantee failure. You might no longer without a doubt pressure to get to a specific location in New York City if you were making plans to strength there, would possibly you?

On the opportunity hand, you may have particular commands in advance than leaving to make sure you arrived at your meant area. The same is going for statements like, "I need to get in higher form," which is probably too favored to be taken drastically.

It has no strain in the back of it, and you could no longer even have the ability to inform if you've succeeded. How so? Technically, you'll be in higher shape now than whilst you began if you surely lost one pound!

Get particular and determine what you really want because of the reality it's far apparent that this might be now not what you had in mind. Consider setting a purpose like, "By the surrender of this year, I want to lose 35 pounds and healthy into the identical pants I wore in college." See the distinction? If you operate specifics like those, you may now be able to determine at the equal time as you arrive at your excursion spot.

Measurable: This complements the idea of retaining your reason measurable, which goes hand in hand with being particular on your assertion. Why does this depend wide range?

Make sure your assertion gives a clear reaction to the question "how plenty" The solution, the usage of the same instance as above, would be 35 pounds.

To maintain you on target, you may pass even further with this. Create smaller milestones which you would love to advantage along the way in desire to without a doubt list your typical intention.

You may say, "I want to lose 35 kilos, because of this I need to lose at least 3 kilos every month for a 12 months."

This gives you a super manner to display your development, as a manner to preserve you inspired. After all, a journey of one thousand miles starts offevolved offevolved with a single step, consistent with an ancient Chinese proverb. In a similar vein, it is not possible to lose 35 pounds all of sudden, however you can do it this week!

Attainable: It is going with out saying which you want to maintain your cause inside the bounds of motive for this one. Expecting to run at the treadmill as soon as and lose 20 kilos in a day is unrealistic. Instead, you need to divide your aim into practicable chunks that are competitive sufficient to maintain you walking difficult but moreover viable.

If now not, you may give up after some weeks of falling brief of your desires. It might be higher initially a decrease reason and increase it as you continuously surpass it each week.

Realistic: Realistic objectives are by using the usage of the usage of definition viable objectives, but there may be a first-class line retaining apart the 2. You won't have the ability or willing to attain a specific benchmark, even though it is probably possible to gain this.

For example, on the same time as decreasing your body fats to 7 percentage can be theoretically bodily feasible, it can no longer be sensible. Your intention want to be to get in affordable form in case you are beginning out as a sofa potato or 100 pounds overweight. Trying to decorate your health from in that you're now to that of a triathlete isn't always certainly sensible, and also you chance putting yourself up for disappointment within the destiny.

The mere reality that some thing is possible (functionality) does not assure that you'll be a hit (practical). So, attempt to maintain your purpose in the middle, and everything ought to exercise for you!

I want to lessen my frame fat percent from 22 to fourteen percent over the route of seven months.

However, maintain in mind that a difficult undertaking is probably made less complex because it will keep you impacted. Setting the bar too low may additionally purpose you to grow to be disinterested. Only you can decide wherein the perfect balance lies, and if you experience together with you want a hint extra motivation in the center, you could constantly beautify your goals!

Time Determined: You've in all likelihood discovered that each instance includes a specific time period. This is important due to the fact with out it, you may not be capable of make on-the-pass plans.

You might most effective need to lose 2 kilos a month if you gave yourself years to lose 50 pounds. You will need to double that amount, notwithstanding the truth that, if your cause is to shed kilos in only three hundred and sixty five days.

Therefore, a essential issue of your purpose is your cut-off date, which wants to be very unique.

Next, what? Now which you have a particular objective in thoughts that you have labored difficult to make compelling, congratulations! What's the subsequent circulate, and the way can you're making the maximum of this? You want to continuously remind your self of this purpose through posting it someplace you may see it each day, as grow to be already said. This will characteristic a reminder of your goals and also can useful aid within the formation of latest workout routines. It best takes 21 days to set up a ultra-current normal or habit, so after 3 weeks of healthful ingesting and exercising, lifestyles can be a good buy much less complicated.

However, if you've battled your weight for a long time, your eating behavior and sedentary way of life may be deeply ingrained in you. To break out of this rut, you will possibly need to be competitive and try some element a touch crazy!

Is a terrible clinical report what finally motivates you to shed kilos? Then show your scientific records, the effects of any blood tests, or honestly a reminder of your horrific state of fitness subsequent for your stated cause.

Why in the world would possibly you engage in any such morbid interest? You see, if you're like most human beings, you'll need to brief overlook approximately about this demanding development. This is simplest natural due to the fact you do no longer want to don't forget uncomfortable subjects all of the time.

But it's far important that you do so because it would encourage you need nothing else in your lifestyles. It becomes clearer to you which you cannot provide you with the cash for to waste this time at the same time as you see the check consequences or your physician's be aware every morning.

Alternatively, you may have a more uplifting cause, which consist of becoming proper right into a smaller get dressed length for a coming close to event. Why no longer submit a image of the contested dress or the real dress itself?

It can also sound a piece out of the normal, however seeing your motive proper in the front of you every day will make it a lot much less hard for you to say no to the donuts at paintings.

The image of that get dressed could be though for your mind while you're tempted to abandon your weight loss plan or skip your workout. Although it is able to appear trustworthy, this really works! Why no longer deliver it a attempt when you preserve in mind which you might in all likelihood begin getting effects which you have never visible earlier than?

Get Support: You may additionally count on that you are done at this detail given that you have created a SMART aim and located it in a prominent region in which you'll see it every day. Although that could be a fantastic starting, you still need one extra aspect to obtain success!

You see, the cause why maximum human beings fail is that they do not installation a guide system to get them via the in fact tough instances. These will necessarily stand up, and somewhere along your non-public weight loss adventure, you may experience like giving up.

It may be as easy as having a difficult day at paintings, discomfort out of your most current day workout, or melancholy making you want to eat a whole chocolate cake! Whatever the scenario, there might be a time at the same time as you require manual to get you thru a tough duration.

Who must you touch to shape your personal assist organisation? It need to skip without announcing that you want a supportive partner in your weight loss efforts. Since they in all likelihood see you every day, it might be best if you could enlist the resource of your associate.

Additionally, you probably percentage as a minimum one meal each day with them, allowing them to take a look at your consuming conduct as nicely. Unfortunately, your associate might not be open to trade or even be adversarial to your weightloss plan. They may be dangerous, but they'll be now not willing to trade, so they will handiest be a terrible have an effect on. If so, you will want extra guide from special pals or own family individuals to make up for the manual you aren't getting at domestic.

In truth, it's miles great to ask a chum who's already physical in shape for assist due to the reality they're aware of what it takes to preserve the load off. Additionally, they won't be tempted to bypass exercising workouts or eat dangerous food, simply so they may not provide in in case you beg them to.

If you do now not recognise absolutely everyone like this, look for a chum with whom you can get in shape so you can art work collectively to shed the kilos. As you can not skip your exercise when you have a assembly at the gymnasium, this can be a sturdy motivator. You may additionally have a further incentive to maintain your diet considering that you'll be required to inform them what you have got been consuming.

Free Personal Training: You can advantage from my enjoy similarly to having a friend or partner as a supply of assist. There, you may see my meal plans and the sports activities I pick out to do. This is just like having a private instructor, but while not having to spend any coins. Additionally, preserve in mind that you can get in touch with me if you have any questions; I'm right right here to make certain you are a success in dropping the burden.

Combining it All: You now understand a way to create a terrific intention a good way to preserve you pretty inspired. Keep your desires precise, measurable, accessible, practical, and time-nice!

You can be capable of efficiently navigate and determine when you have arrived at your holiday spot if all of those conditions are met. Then, absolutely glance at it once a day or more to keep your new intention sparkling. The next step is to enlist the help of your associate or a near pal that will help you stay on course each time you are tempted to stray. You may be in a outstanding position to gain your weight loss dreams if all of those factors come into play.

How Diets Work

Losing weight is easy; Simply eat fewer calories every day than your frame desires to feature to shed pounds.

It is going with out pronouncing that we devour due to the truth it is crucial for our our our bodies to feature. We will placed on weight if we devour more than we want. Consider this: an growth in each day caloric intake of just 3 hundred electricity have to bring about a 20-pound weight advantage over the path of a one year! We are consuming greater power than we need, so this would be a remarkable strength stability.

Going in advance, keep in mind a eating regimen as a feeding technique in that you can modify your calorie consumption. One approach you can use to shed pounds is to devour fewer electricity. Don't allow the fact that culmination and veggies are wholesome fool you into thinking you could munch on they all day. The contrary is real, as you could see. Keep in mind that big calorie intake is what sincerely counts. Still, those substances contain strength. You can select the meals you need to eat and calculate how many electricity you need based totally completely on your weight reduction desires using my meal planner.

Many humans expect they may not be hungry because of the truth they notably reduced the variety of strength on their feeding plan. This should seem. However, the hunger pangs can be decreased if you may consume every 2-four hours.

Divide the amount of hours you're conscious with the aid of 3 to get a quick technique. If you spend 15 hours an afternoon wakeful, five food want to be your target. Using my meal planner, it become decided which you required 1500 power substantial, or an average of 3 hundred power regular with meal, for the day. Your possibilities of fulfillment boom manner to this meal planner.

A meal replacement let you stay on course if you get busy at art work and are not capable of consume a meal. Due to the unpredictable nature of lifestyles, I do use those often all through the week.

I do now not advise skipping any meals at the start of your dietary plan due to the truth doing so may also result in what I communicate to as "compensating." In essence, because of the truth you skipped a meal, you'll probable overeat at your subsequent meal psychologically. This will necessarily result in progressed meals intake and weight benefit.

Diets normally fail due to the truth they're too restrictive for optimum people. Don't suppose that every one you want to do is eat water and eat veggies all day. No, that may not paintings over the prolonged haul.

With my meal planner, you calculate your calorie consumption and then create a weekly menu based totally at the substances you experience eating, now not what a few food regimen expert says you should consume.

A meal planner allows many people via doing away with the guesswork worried in identifying the right meals they ought to devour an terrific manner to shed pounds. What can I devour? Is the maximum not unusual question I gather with regards to weight reduction. It is now feasible to answer to this question.

Rule of thumb

One of the crucial component components to sticking to a diet plan is region. It can take months or perhaps years to shed pounds through a right diet plan and get in your excellent weight. Yo-yo diet can result from any immoderate diet that encourages short results. Yo-yo eating regimen is the exercise of dropping weight whilst adhering to a eating regimen, only to in the end overeat and advantage lower again the load out of place.

This takes area due to the fact the weight-reduction plan he observed end up excessively restrictive, banning many food organizations and seriously proscribing his meals consumption. He can not stick with this healthy eating plan, so he offers in and eats extra. Or it might be the result of a lack of challenge as fast as the famous weight has been reached. This is normally what happens even as you observe a really excessive-calorie food regimen.

In order to save you that, you need to adopt a wholesome lifestyle and learn how to consume well, exercising regularly, and get sufficient sleep. It may be difficult inside the starting to interrupt terrible conduct. But in case you observe your new eating method for at the least 21 to 30 days, it should lay a solid foundation for success.

Your large special will need to useful resource you as you switch from an unstable food regimen to a healthful one. I've seen it arise a long way too frequently in which the person who is closest to you may undermine your efforts. Why now not persuade them to accept your new feeding method? Making this variation may additionally have a high-quality effect on their fitness however the fact that they do not need to lose weight.

The truth that my meal planner has limitless feasible mixtures is the very last reason why the usage of one is important for success. How do I anticipate you to stay on fowl and broccoli every day once I realize I could not? You won't lose interest because of the shape of food to be had, collectively with food you experience, and your opportunities of fulfillment can be notably progressed.

Just maintain in thoughts that you can get lower back on the right track the next day if you fall off the wagon and devour one or extra meals that exceed your every day calorie restriction. In the end, all this is required of you is compliance ninety% of the time. Obviously, you can not do this every day, however doing it once each week may not notably limit your attempts to lose weight.

Trade Secrets

The weight loss business enterprise is maintaining a number of of factors from you and doesn't want you to apprehend them. They are promoting fads, devices, and drugs to folks which can be determined to lose weight, and their enterprise is booming as a end result.

Unfortunately, people's wallets are commonly the first-rate detail that is getting lighter. Only a small part of those who purchase into the sort of techniques without a doubt attain dropping weight and keeping it off. Many of those methods are vain.

A few of these commercial business enterprise secrets and techniques are as follows:

The majority of classified ads for weight reduction merchandise deceive the client. The large majority of weight reduction products that you pay interest about at the radio and be aware on infomercials do not even art work as promised. Nevertheless, the ones merchandise are advertised to clients with claims collectively with "Lose the weight and hold it off," "Eat some factor you want," and "no weight loss plan or exercising required." In famous, if something appears too right to be authentic, it likely is.

It does not continuously propose a few element works truely because it's "scientifically examined" or "physician endorsed." These claims also are common, but they by no means reveal the area or authors of the studies so that you can independently take a look at their validity.

What does it without a doubt advocate, then? These "fitness professionals" frequently have a financial stake within the product, simply so they maximum probable surpassed over the clinical research. Even if it end up reviewed, they might not have adhered to low-priced assessment necessities. Why would you need to perform a little problem like that and hazard your health?

A product's protection for clients or capability to stay as much as its guarantees aren't guaranteed sincerely due to the fact the government lets in it to be presented. There is a brilliant misconception that the authorities would possibly forbid a product from entering the marketplace if it might endanger you. People frequently recollect that the authorities need to first pre-approve them, but this isn't always commonly the case.

The protection of merchandise advertised as "herbal" or "herbal" can't be assured. The perception that a product want to be secure definitely because it includes herbal factors is some other commonplace misconception. However, businesses are loose to release their products onto the marketplace up till the FDA receives evidence that a product is risky.

You need to not do not forget the whole lot you pay attention because of the reality it could no longer be real. You should keep away from products that make grandiose claims because of the reality there are various available that absolutely do no longer live as a good deal as their claims.

Likewise, do not accept as true with the claims made through fad diets. Anything that calls for abrupt and drastic changes to your ingesting conduct can be very tough to hold through the years.

They'll start you on a short weight loss cycle, that is constantly determined with the aid of a period at some point of which, in a few instances, you can advantage all of the weight you misplaced plus some as soon as your regular consuming styles resume.

Additionally, it makes it even harder the subsequent time you try to lose the weight. These diets don't have any immoderate fine effects on health, and do you in reality take delivery of as genuine with that there is probably a call for for emblem spanking new ones in the event that they did?

Additionally, you need to not rely on the cash-decrease decrease lower back assure. The danger of getting your cash back is ready equal to the chance that the product will stay as an entire lot as its ensures.

Additionally, there isn't a magic therapy or short repair on the manner to permit you to eventually shed pounds. You can nearly in reality guarantee that if a product makes such claims, they might not be true.

Chapter 2: What Should I Do Now?

You ought to be dedicated to any weight loss program so that you can be positive at it. Only with the aid of adopting the right thoughts-set are you able to reap fulfillment. Before you could go with the flow without delay to the following segment of your weight loss program, you ought to first prepare yourself with the aid of the use of way of knowledge what level you're in. It won't be visible, but it's miles although gift.

Pre-contemplation is the initial level: You do not do not forget your self as overweight. You don't enjoy like altering who you are. You might not ask for assist besides there is a lot of pressure. But if that occurred, you'll no longer offer in; you would without a doubt surrender, feeling defeated via manner of your very private situation.

The 2nd is mirrored photograph: This is the thing at which you admit that you have a weight problem and start to keep in mind a solution. However, you are unwilling to enforce that treatment. Knowing what steps to take to impact a exchange, however in no manner being prepared to obtain this, you may surely don't forget it. You will put off enforcing the answer.

The zero.33 is planning: You've sooner or later made up your mind to deal with your weight hassle. You forestall residing to your trouble and start figuring out the solution. Additionally, you will start to envision a time within the destiny while you are thinner and experience hundreds higher. However, you aren't but truely dedicated at this issue. Even so, you will likely however be on the fence approximately the solution because it calls for a life-style adjustment.

Action is the fourth: You start to take steps toward losing weight. You may additionally begin making food options and attractive in daily exercising. It is the first step in the route of achieving your particular aim. Setting goals is a need to at the same time as looking for to shed pounds. It's very possibly that your complete healthy dietweight-reduction plan may not circulate as you had was hoping in case you do not set your dreams.

Describe the subsequent:

•What is your present day-day situation proper now? In order to shed pounds, make a listing of all your eating behavior, meals options, and other factors. Exercising, and so on.

•What motivates your desire to shed kilos? This is probably for a forthcoming event, the summer time, or maybe for a completely unique someone. Write down the one, largest motive that includes mind.

•What benefits do you benefit from dropping weight? As many as you can listing. Health, more strength, a accomplice's admiration, and so on. Are some examples. This want to be your primary using pressure.

•Your Objective. Write this in ambitious to help it in fact stick to your mind: "I want to lose XX pounds of weight in XX days."

Personally, I expect it is unrealistic to set a motive of more than 10 kilos each weeks, specially if you're searching for to achieve it for the primary time. Be realistic. You need to apply the verb "want" rather than "wish."

Record the whole lot on paper, then assessment it often. Placing it wherein you can see it's going to assist. You might be continuously reminded of WHY you try this and what the blessings are once you begin seeing it every day.

Once you start, do no longer give up because it could not be clean.

Stepping Out of Your Comfort Zone

Consider your motivation for now not simply searching for to shed kilos if you find out yourself springing up with justifications in vicinity of STARTING an green food plan. You must very own the functionality to push beyond your consolation sector and, in the phrases of Nike's catchphrase, "JUST DO IT!"

Maintenance can be the closing step. You ought to maintain the momentum you had in the route of the movement degree. If at any factor you stop being dedicated or supportive, you may revert to any of the sooner degrees.

The final degree of your diet regime is therefore the most vital due to the truth you want to hold your dedication over an prolonged term. There are severa techniques you may rent to maintain your determination.

Make a list of your preliminary motivations for doing this earlier than anything else. To maintain your popularity for your desires, overview the listing every day. Avoid thinking a few component negative. Never use phrases like "in no manner" or "depriving" to your vocabulary. You are first-class having desserts "on occasion and punctiliously" in choice to "in no way." As a quit result, the phrase "deprived" may be changed to "choosing" even as you recollect that you have determined to forego chocolate cakes.

Imagine on your mind's eye a slimmer model of yourself wearing out all of the things you have continuously favored. Your electricity of mind to live with this plan and be determined to be successful might be boosted with the useful resource of this visualization. Every day, on every occasion you awaken and every time you sense your dedication waning, carry out this visualization.

Who to Approach When You Want to Lose Weight?

You need to involve some other human beings on your weight reduction journey now which you've made the decision to shed kilos. These human beings will let you in a variety of strategies, along with deciding on a healthy eating plan approach, organising goals, and offering you with motivation as you circulate in advance.

A dietician: A dietician have to have a extensive base of know-how that might help you in know-how your frame and making ready a diet plan an awesome way to satisfy your individual desires due to the truth, within the majority of states and nations, obtaining a scientific license is a prerequisite for turning into a dietician. Meal planners are a much much less highly-priced preference to dieticians. My meal planner is a progressive new device that has a patent pending. It assists you in building genuinely balanced diets using your favored meals via taking walks with you as even though they were your personal personal dietician or nutritionist.

An man or woman teacher: Most humans have by no means been taught a way to workout well. This, for my part, could be very crucial in case you've never engaged in any form of weight training. I wouldn't sign an prolonged-time period settlement with a teacher, and I'd want them to recognize my desires and the manner they plan to assist me in reaching them. I might caution you that for at least the first three hundred and sixty five days, you need to scale the exercises in terms of weight and duration.

Family and buddies: I constantly dislike doing this, but I actually have a plan that I receive as true with you can located to use rapid.

I detested telling humans whenever I released into considered one in every of my a hundred diets. Because this changed into but every different food regimen I come to be beginning, I notion they have been judging me. Instead, say (inside the occasion that they ask) that you're definitely in search of to eat a chunk more healthy and that you're completed with diets while you are at the dinner desk throughout a party, tour, or distinct specific event.

Persisting Through Failure

You will always fail even as seeking to shed kilos or maintain it off due to the fact you are best human. People who're successful at dropping weight did no longer give up while subjects have been given difficult; alternatively, they continued and located a lesson.

The crucial strategies for coping with failure are to Keep attempting and selecting topics up.

Don't fear about the little matters in case you stray from your food regimen or pass an workout day. Don't permit it to stop you. Get it from your head. Consider all of your correct days in location of in reality one mistake. The more healthful life-style alternatives you're making, the greater right days you have; earlier than you apprehend it, the horrific days are few and far amongst. But the secret is to persevere and get through the tough instances. Consider it a cheat day, then pass on. This is how you persist; it's far ok to fail for a day, in reality do not permit it emerge as each week, then a month.

To deal with disasters, you should learn how to take transport of them as a herbal a part of life.

The next step is to take education from your mistakes. It is frequently greater effective to analyze from your errors than from your successes.

When you fail, view it as a training moment. Just like in business organization, even as you strive a few element and fail, you research what does no longer work.

The identical holds proper for losing weight. Perhaps you need to abstain from consuming if you find that whenever you drink, your new food plan suffers. Reschedule your exercising if you find out which you continuously bypass it on Fridays because of a past due paintings meeting.

Along with loss of life and taxes, failure is a given in existence. Even if you may, you wouldn't need to because you can't avoid it. Your failures and successes both teach you precious instructions approximately lifestyles. Don't be scared of failing; simply maintain attempting and keep learning.

Buddy System

Adding some obligation to your normal is one of the first rate topics you can do while looking for to lose weight. How do you skip about that?

The Buddy System

A wonderful motivator is having a pal with whom to strive weight loss. When you in reality tell a person approximately your weight loss dreams, you'll enjoy more chargeable for attaining them. They also may be beneficial because of the truth the individual can recognize your problems with weight loss. You can inspire every different with the useful resource of way of sharing each your victories and your setbacks.

A exercising accomplice is beneficial in case you exercise regularly. They can transform a stupid jog or stroll proper right into a treatment session that also serves as workout. Bringing a chum along for a hike within the wasteland is constantly extra exciting!

Having a chum is likewise useful if you revel in weightlifting. You guys can push every fantastic on the equal time as additionally encouraging and assisting each different out with such things as spots on heavy lifts.

The sad truth is that you can possibly find out a weight loss friend on your circle of buddies nowadays. Don't worry in case you can not; you could always do it definitely on-line.

The bottom line is that operating with a pal can help with responsibility, useful resource, and motivation if you're looking for to shed pounds. Now move discover your weight loss associate!

Why It's Important to keep a Daily Schedule

Setting up a every day training time desk is the subsequent step in making plans your weight loss desires. Personally, I discover that 6AM is a extremely good time for me.

It become hard to rouse so early at the begin, however in the long run it became a dependancy. I'll list some advantages of workout currently of day.

1) You have finished your each day exercise.

2) You have the afternoon loose to spend collectively in conjunction with your own family, companion, friends, and so forth.

three) It's k if you aren't on time at art work due to the truth your workout is already finished.

But the ones are the reasons I educate at this hour of the morning. Friends of mine have admitted to favoring the late afternoon and early midnight. Once greater, the time does now not truely count range as loads due to the fact the fact which you need to finish the undertaking.

Maintaining Your Balance: You're more likely to paste in your desires when you have a difficult and rapid time table to comply with, so record the whole thing in a magazine or different journaling tool like a cellphone. However, if you do pass a exercising or have a further snack, you can be aware it and remedy to do better the following time.

Understanding Your Daily Routine: It can assist to have a written time desk of whilst you have to workout or devour your meals so you are organized. In this manner you can time desk subjects around your exercise times, in vicinity of scheduling over them and surely lacking sports activities altogether.

This is easy to do, and whilst you begin doing it, you may find out that you leave out your exercise workouts greater often until you clearly lose track of your fitness desires.

Lose More Weight: By sticking to a schedule, you are more likely to complete your workout routines on time and ultimately lose extra weight (or very, only a few in the long run).

You will find out it heaps more hard to keep a regular rate of weight loss in case you frequently transfer among diets, pass exercises, or skip meals, which confuses your frame's metabolism.

Chapter 3: Healthy Nutrition And Its Benefits

You can also have heard a whole lot of humans say that consuming a healthy eating regimen is essential for preserving a wholesome body, but you want to recognize what healthy vitamins in reality includes and why it is so important. Define nutrients first.

"Nutrition is the method of giving your body all the critical vitamins a excellent manner to allow it to increase in a healthful and balanced way."

This is the only definition of nutrients, and it informs you that you need to devour healthful foods which might be rich in critical nutrients. Your frame can grow to be sturdy and healthful with right nutrition, and it is able to moreover broaden and heal on its own. While a horrible nutrients plan can weaken your frame, make you ill, and prevent you from combating off a few minor ailments.

Calories In - Calories Out

Most people who want to shed pounds have experimented with a whole lot of diets, dietary supplements, and/or plans. There are many awesome weight loss strategies that can be sold. They're all making outrageous claims.

The harsh truth is that there aren't any magic pills, diets, or exercise device in an effort to make weight vanish in a single day. It all comes all of the manner right down to eating properly, preserving best fitness, and consuming fewer energy than you dissipate.

That is the start location of the proverb "electricity in, power out." Make sure you deplete extra strength (out) than you are taking in (in).

This is a naive way of questioning, and a healthful diet plan includes greater than just counting energy. We'll take a look at that in later chapters, but for now, permit's interest on setting up a calorie deficit.

You'll want a few essential records to track this. You should first decide what number of power you manifestly burn each day. It all comes proper right down to things like weight and age.

How to Determine How Many Calories You Burn Each Day

Men's BMR calculation (kg) BMR is calculated as follows: sixty six.Five + thirteen.Seventy five x weight in kg + 5.003 x peak in cm - (6.755 x age in years)

Men's BMR calculation (pounds) BMR is calculated as follows: sixty six + 6.23 x weight in pounds + 12.7 x peak in inches - (6.76 x age in years)

Female BMR calculation (kg) BMR is calculated as follows: 655.1 + (9.563 x weight in kg) + 1.850 x pinnacle in cm - (four.676 x age in years)

BMR for women is calculated as follows: BMR = 655 + four.35 times weight in kilos + 4.7

times pinnacle in inches - (four.7 x age in years)

This equation will display you what number of electricity you burn every day truely from respiratory, heartbeat, and so on. These are the calories you'll burn if you remained table sure all day (basal metabolic fee).

Once you apprehend that determine, you want to start maintaining song of the electricity you devour and burn. There is a lot of statistics to maintain tune of, which makes this challenging. It's no longer about ravenous yourself or strolling out nonstop till you bypass out. It all comes proper all the manner down to being conscious of what you located into and exert out of your body. Even in spite of the truth that losing weight can be difficult, if you could manipulate your consumption and expenditure of energy, you will be a success!

Clean Eating

The critical weight loss precept, energy in versus energy out, has already been discussed. It is a important tip due to the truth you continue to need to be careful about in which you have become your energy from. It's probable not a notable concept to eat corndogs in step with day so you can lessen your calorie consumption.

Although there can be no reputable definition for the phrase "consuming easy," it commonly refers to consuming entire, healthy meals and averting processed meals and delicate sugars.

While it can no longer continuously be feasible to consume first-rate "easy" meals, when you have grow to be the bulk of your energy from the ones food, you are doing awesome.

Fast food and junk meals are mechanically eliminated out of your diet on the same time as you consume smooth due to the reality you keep away from processed meals. Don't worry if you eat some processed meals; the purpose is to consume as little of it as feasible.

Here are a few preferred pointers for consuming healthy:

Read labels cautiously: Read the additives and nutritional information on each product you purchase.

every time viable, pick out out whole grains: Whole grain does now not normally equate to entire wheat, each!

Frequently devour culmination and greens: They are fantastic assets of healthful whole electricity.

Don't purchase microwaveable food, consume out lots less, and put together greater of your very very personal meals. Even though they're marketed as "wholesome," the ones food may be very immoderate in sodium.

When cooking, pick out lean meats: It's good enough to devour meat due to the truth the protein will help you enjoy glad and assemble muscle. Excellent meat options encompass fish and hen.

Steer clean of processed meats like hot dogs and bologna.

Whole nuts which might be unsalted or lightly salted can take the region of junk food.

Visit these loose net web sites for fantastic smooth recipes: http://easy-stir-fry-recipes.Com and http://low-carb-chickenrecipes.Com

Don't fear about slacking off; allow yourself the occasional cheat day.

It may be difficult to eat healthily whilst out, however more eateries are starting to provide this option. If you're in reality hungry, you may probably want to characteristic some protein to a salad, despite the fact that!

A outstanding way to make sure which you are wholesome common and which you shed pounds is to eat cleanly. You do now not should attempt to reveal on a transfer and make the transition in a single day, but it isn't always clean. Clean up your weight loss plan in case you're intense about losing weight and enhancing your health.

Water Is Your Best Friend

According to analyze, you need to drink as a minimum 8 glasses of water each day, but how an entire lot you really need will rely upon your weight. Your weight could want to be divided via 2. Therefore, someone weighing 100 eighty pounds have to require 90 ouncesOf water steady with day.

So why is water endorsed through manner of specialists and why is it belief to be so vital to living a healthy life?

First off, it aids within the removal of waste products, which prevents dehydration and continues the kidneys' appropriate health. Additionally, it helps to rush up metabolism, which aids in weight reduction.

But further to paying attention to what specialists advise, you need to prioritize taking note of your body. Naturally, you can drink water to rehydrate yourself at the equal time as you are thirsty.

Depending on the sort of paintings you do, you must try to develop the dependancy of regularly ingesting water or, even better, keeping a water bottle available. This is especially crucial on pretty heat days because the warmth motives you to perspire and your body loses water, so you will want to rehydrate.

Water has a vital feature in our lives due to this. In addition to having no energy, it is also the terrific and healthiest manner to quench your thirst. In the long time, you might think about converting fruit liquids and sodas with water at every meal to assist reduce your calorie consumption. You'll moreover revel in lots higher with out the extra sugar that consists of the opportunity liquids.

Chapter 4: The Importance Of Exercise

In this monetary damage I'm going to tell you what works excellent for melting fats like butter on a heat variety.

Exercising

First of all, the human body is constructed for movement. Exercise has many benefits besides the apparent ones of retaining a healthy body weight.

1) Fights infection;

2) Elevates your temper;

3) Increases your strength;

4) Aids in higher sleep; and

5) Better sex as well

Seven out of ten adults, or almost 4 out of ten, are not physical energetic on a regular foundation, consistent with a current survey. You run the hazard of growing coronary coronary heart sickness, diabetes, and stroke in case you do no longer exercise. About three hundred,000 people have died due to this.

You want to talk with a health practitioner earlier than starting an exercising application. If you have got been sitting on the couch and no longer jogging out for a while, that is important.

There are many superb perspectives on fat loss inside the global these days. Running is generally the primary exercise interest people do. In any case, it will growth your coronary coronary heart charge and is likewise aerobic.

What burns the most fats is cardio exercising, proper? You is probably surprised to analyze that walking isn't always in truth that effective at burning fat. That's because of the fact as soon as your frame has turn out to be conditioned with the useful resource of the exercising, you regularly obtain a plateau (Peele, 2010).

In assessment, I've determined a way that guarantees you in no manner plateau by means of frequently growing the wishes with each exercise. Additionally, it burns fat up to 3,000% more successfully than your morning run!

Why HIIT is Better Than Running

It is an specific approach and is known as HIIT, or High Intensity Interval Training. It will reduce the length of your exercising workouts and expend to 9 instances greater fats than taking walks (Cossaboon). That way it is 36 instances extra effective regular while combined with the fact that it completes in 1 / four the time. How is this even feasible?

First off, you burn extra energy because of the intensity of the exercising itself. You pop out in advance notwithstanding the truth that a smaller aspect of these come honestly from fat due to the truth the whole is higher.

The maximum amazing element of HIIT schooling is, however, the second way it features. Your metabolism is improved for as a exquisite deal as 24 hours after your exercise is over. That manner that on the same time as you are lounging to your couch at eleven p.M. The equal night time, you can be burning fats!

HIIT emerge as a excellent suit for me because of the reality I cost getting the most out of my cash. Additionally, you nice want to workout three times steady with week to start seeing effects; you do now not even want to exercising every day.

How Does it Work?

The HIIT technique employs a two-pronged technique to supply consequences fast. You will use exquisite intensities sooner or later of your exercise in preference to preserving one intensity the whole time.

Running at a first rate pace is a exceptional example of the number one, that could be a slight stage. The 2nd is brief bursts of excessive intensity, like sprinting at your pinnacle tempo.

You must train at a slower tempo for two to five minutes, observed by using manner of a brief burst of excessive depth exercise lasting 10 to thirty seconds. Repeat this template over again while returning to the mild stage at the same time as 15 to 20 minutes have passed.

Your metabolism could be in overdrive at the perception, and it is able to stay that way for severa hours or perhaps the relaxation of the day. This manner that at the equal time as you exercise and at the identical time as your body is recovering in a while, you are both burning fat. This will accelerate your outcomes and start melting the fat off of your body proper away.

Stay In the Zone

But in case you do no longer hold your coronary coronary heart rate up immoderate enough at some point of your fats loss routine, you may not enjoy any of these awesome benefits.

What price want to you goal for to get the most out of HIIT? Your coronary coronary coronary heart charge ought to be close to your safe restrict at a few stage in the quick times even as you're working as hard as you could.

How can you return to this conclusion? First, subtract your age from 220 to determine your most coronary heart price. Then, even as you are inside the immoderate depth a part of your HIIT session, you have to purpose for eighty 5% of this range (Baker, 2011).

To hit the beats in step with minute required to provide the popular effect, you may want to paintings more tough than you in all likelihood don't forget. You have no longer labored yourself tough sufficient if you could however speak on the identical time as doing this or if you are not gasping for air in some time.

Melt the Fat Away

You'll have a robust device to beneficial resource you in your weight-reduction plan whilst you operate HIIT on the aspect of your purpose heart charge. Incorporating this kind of workout into your fat loss ordinary will hasten your development and beautify your consequences!

Since HIIT allows you to transport even further than conventional aerobic schooling, it's far a greater powerful technique for burning fats. You see, the quick durations of excessive exercising are designed to push you close to your restrict whenever.

Since you cannot preserve this degree all through a exercising, your electricity expenditure will necessarily drop.

For example, you is probably able to sprint at your pinnacle pace for ten to 15 seconds, but now not for the whole thirty minute exercise. You ought to sluggish all of the manner right down to a quick run to get via the exercising, which has particular consequences to your body.

Add Kettlebell Strength Training to Your Routine

Strength schooling with kettlebells is a useful complement in your HIIT sports activities. Women avoid the burden room, even as many guys rush to the health club. You also can accept as actual with that doing this form of exercise will make you look bulky and muscle-sure in choice to provide you with the lean look you desire.

However, weight lifting with kettlebells might be very effective for weight loss whilst accomplished nicely. You will keep your flexibility at the same time as furthermore growing lean muscle with the exercising I've covered, offering you with a nice athletic appearance.

In addition to being outstanding for exclusive reasons, load-bearing exercising has been confirmed to save you osteoporosis (Rogers, 2012). For your decrease body, you may gain this advantage with the aid of manner of truly strolling, however on your higher body, you must boom weights to acquire the same bone-constructing results.

Additionally, resistance education can growth your metabolism for numerous hours following your exercise, in case you want to further your weight loss efforts. Women ought to utilize the weight room and the super kettlebell to the fullest so you can advantage all of those advantages.

Why Use a Kettlebell for Exercise? A right question. I did now not actually apprehend it the primary time I observed a person train with one. But after being requested to participate in a exercise, I end up able to recognize just how beneficial those little guidelines may be for getting into form.

Unless you have been living in a give way Afghanistan, you have likely heard that kettlebells are Russian in beginning place and that the fitness industry has welcomed them with open hands.

Let's speak about the numerous blessings of training with kettlebells:

•Strengthening and muscular endurance

•No health club club is crucial;

•you could education consultation interior or outdoor;

•you may burn fat and shed kilos;

•you could construct lean muscle;

•you can growth mental durability;

•you can expand a strong center and appealing abs.

Choosing the Right Kettlebell

When starting any kettlebell workout software, that may be a crucial choice. Women need to start with an 18-pound kettlebell and men with a 35-pound bell. In the start those weights have to get you off at the right foot and at the same time as the workout workouts are finished with the right intensity they're masses heavy.

Security First

I've said it in advance than, however it's far essential which you communicate collectively along with your medical doctor in advance than starting any bodily health routine. Despite the kettlebell's relative "lightness," the use of it incorrectly can despite the fact that result in damage. It's also crucial to warmth up nicely in advance than beginning any of the sporting sports activities on this e-book. Start out slowly and get familiar with the basics.

Footwear

When using a kettlebell, it's miles vital to preserve your toes flat on the ground continually. Wearing "walking" shoes with a raised heel is not suggested. You would possibly in all likelihood get hurt in case you do not stand successfully due to this. To shop a couple of bucks, you may wear minimalist footwear or surely skip barefoot.

Getting higher with exercising

I appreciate your choice to get started out out education and your strength of mind to paintings closer to getting the frame you deserve. But for the number one week, the best element I need you to do is watch the films that go along with it; after that, I really need you to exercise the kettlebell swing.

The swing is the most crucial waft that I even though paintings on, and at the same time as I do now not cause for perfection, I do try and maintain proper shape.

You can find my endorsed kettlebell exercising in the following financial smash. This is entire with pictures and recommendations for wearing out every day's exercise.

Kettlebell Workout Routine

No depend if you've ever used a kettlebell or now not, ensure to select out a weight that you could bypass with out getting harm. Kettlebells are an great device for getting into form, but they want to be treated with care.

You will see results from this workout after eight weeks in case you have a look at a healthy weight-reduction plan and get sufficient rest. Prior to starting any exercise software, make certain to get your clinical health practitioner's approval.

The workout is meant to be finished four days in line with week. Mon./Tues., Wednesday as a rest day, and then Thursday/Friday are my recommendations. Life takes place, of direction. As intently as you could, look at the plan.

Each exercise's define is supplied underneath, followed by way of manner of using extra thorough instructions.

Front Plank

The beginning characteristic is in your palms and knees with the lower back flat. Contract the belly muscle mass. Without rotating the trunk or sagging or arching the backbone, growth yourself into the frenzy up characteristic on the side of your weight to your forearms and feet. Keep your head up looking ahead. The aim is to keep this function for 60 seconds. If you can't keep for 1 minute, then repeat until 1 minute has elapsed. Continue to respire on the same time as conducting this exercise.

The Hip Flexor Stretch

Movement:

1. Start with left knee on the ground, and right leg up with each palms over head.

2. Hold for about 10 seconds.

3. Switch to the other factor and hold for 10 seconds.

Note: This warmth-up exercising promotes stretching out the center, hip flexors, decrease again, quadriceps, lats, and is absolutely an trendy outstanding stretch to lighten up. This is probable the notable not unusual stretch you could do earlier than any physical occasion.

Push-Up

I realise most human beings assume they recognize a way to perform a push-up.

Movement:

1. Bend the elbows, reducing your body until your pinnacle palms are parallel with the floor.

2. Fully expand your fingers just so your elbows are "locked" out.

The secret is to in fact boom inside the up function together together with your hands locked out. Secondly, make certain that whilst you're in the down feature your fingers are parallel to the floor. Don't suppose fast right here, do them gradual and managed for entire effect of this movement.

Variation: If you are not able to perform a push-up as illustrated, anticipate a stance for your knees to perform them correctly. This is a herbal improvement.

Kettlebell Swing

Movement:

1. Squat down collectively along side your lower once more right now and lift up the load. Don't confuse this with a vertical lower back, actually hold it at once. Don't round your lower back.

2. Squat up and stand erect in conjunction with your shoulders once more.

three. Think sit lower back in vicinity of dip down.

four. Ensure that your hips are prolonged as well as your knees on the top collectively with your frame in a directly line.

five. For the Russian style swing illustrated right here the bell must in no manner pass above parallel.

6. Ensure which you are both barefoot or wearing a minimalist shoe so you are flat footed.

Precautions: Work with light weight first of all till you may carry out the movement efficaciously.

Turkish Get-Up

Movement:

1.Use every of your arms whilst in a fetal function to raise the kettlebell from the ground on the begin of the motion and on the crowning glory of the motion.

2.Next you want to set the foot and hand. Notice that the arm at the kettlebell aspect is vertical with a instantly wrist. The knee on the element of the kettlebell is bent to put together you for in the end reputation up. Both the lats and your middle are engaged and ready for artwork. The arm opposite the kettlebell is located forty five ranges and your opposite leg is straight away.

3.Lock your elbow and hold it locked for the duration of the motion.

four.Keep your shoulder in a "packed" function constantly at some point of the motion.

five.Get up easily and slowly and cope with each characteristic.

6.This isn't an exercising executed swiftly.

Precaution: This appears deceivingly clean. Use a totally mild weight (5lbs) or perhaps a sneaker until you hit every position. In my Hardstyle Kettlebell Certification direction, we used the sneaker. I rather advise the sneaker.

Deadlift

Movement:

1. Straddle the bell together with your ft a piece wider than shoulder-width.

2. Squat down with arms prolonged downward amongst your legs and snatch the bell's cope with with every palms.

three. Ensure that your shoulders are over the bell and maintain your lower returned without delay.

four. Pull the bell off the ground with the aid of extending your hips and knees ensuring your chest is up.

5. Lower the bell on the identical time as squatting down and maintaining your once more taunt with a vertical again.

Precaution: Ensure you do not round your lower back. Ensure you may do an air squat and not using a weight properly in advance than adding any weight.

Snatch

Movement:

1. Begin with the Russian Style swing.

2. Catch the bell softly without "banging" the bell for your wrist.

three. You can try this by the use of "punching" to the pinnacle of the motion.

4. When you lock out on the pinnacle, your arm must be diploma together along side your head.

5. Lower the bell down to finish a swing and repeat as wanted.

Precaution: Keep once more right now, art work with a weight you can correctly control.

Learning the Rack

Movement:

1. Pick up the bell with 1 hand

2. Use your second hand to get the bell into function

three. Now you're within the rack role or in which the clean sooner or later eventually finally ends up

4. Drop the bell down with the useful resource of shifting your hips backwards and "sitting down"

5. The bell is moving simply vertically down through the use of manner of moving your hips again and now not pushing the bell ahead.

Precaution: Keep your back proper away, use a weight that is lighter until you have got a observe the movement.

The Rack

Movement:

1.Stand over the kettlebells. Take a deep breath and hold and pull lower again amongst legs.

2.As the kettlebells come another time (breathe in), bend barely at the knees, pushing your hips backwards allowing the kettlebells to skip amongst your legs. Ensure another time is without delay.

3.Using your glutes like a rubber band, open your hips and propel the bell in advance. As you drive through collectively together with your hips (breathe out) till you return to a triple extension. The bells want to land amongst your arms and forearms, with elbow tucked in some unspecified time inside the future of pass.

four.Your bells are honestly in a racked function.

Precaution: Ensure your once more is instantly, and select out a weight this is inside your ability to soundly bring the weight.

Double Kettlebell Front Squat

Movement:

1. Begin with the bells within the racked role.

2. Set handles really above your collar bone.

3. Have your toes a touch wider than shoulder-width aside.

four. Inhale as you're taking a seat down whilst keeping your lower once more without delay.

five. Exhale on the manner up and stand tall.

Precautions: Do now not round your lower lower back. Ensure your lower lower again is immediately. Select a weight you may as it should be float.

Clean

Movement:

1. Straddle the bell along side your ft a touch greater than shoulder width aside.

2. Your elbow should be part of your torso.

3. Your hips will do all the paintings.

4. Make the bell tour in a at once line; that is the shortest distance amongst 2 devices.

5. Do no longer dip your knees at the same time as receiving or "racking" the bell.

6. Avoid banging your wrist or forearm.

Precautions: Back immediately, choose a weight that you may paintings with well.

Press

Movement:

1. Stand together together with your toes slightly wider than shoulder width.

2. Take the bell from the rack or clean it from the floor and function within the the front of chest with the bell in the direction of the outside of your arm.

three. Press the bell up till your arm is actually extended overhead.

4. Lower to the the the front of your chest.

Precaution: Ensure that you are the usage of a weight with a purpose to permit you carry out the drift nicely.

Overhead or Waiters Walk

Movement:

1. Begin with the bell within the press out position.

2. Ensure that your shoulder and elbow are in a "locked" characteristic.

3. Begin strolling.

Precautions: Make sure you have got a smooth direction (manifestly), pick out out out your weight cautiously

Suitcase Carry

Movement:

1. Pick up the bell as you would a suitcase deadlift in advance than wearing.

2. Keep the shoulders degree and middle tight with out a repayment from one element to three different.

3. A heavier weight may be required to accumulate the popular effect.

Precautions: Ensure you your once more is immediately and now not rounded at the identical time as picking up or placing down the weight. As commonly, choose out a weight you could circulate thoroughly.

Rack Walk

Movement:

1. Begin with the bells in the racked feature.

2. Ensure that the handles are above your collar bones.

3. Keep the bells next on your bicep.

four. Do now not allow the bells slump or sag.

five. Start walking.

Precautions: Ensure your on foot direction is freed from boundaries and select out out a weight you may safely circulate with.

Goblet Squat

Movement:

1. Grab the bell with the aid of the horns.

2. Feet shoulder width apart or a chunk more than shoulder width aside.

three. Pull yourself down.

4. Keep your chest up at the same time as retaining your lower lower back as without delay as possible.

5. Elbows come inner your knees with the burden on your heels and not ft.

6. Stand straight away up.

Precautions: Do no spherical the all over again and pick a weight appropriate in your competencies.

Single Arm Deadlift

Movement:

1. Performed like deadlift but with weight in your facet.

2. Bell might be even together in conjunction with your ankle.

three. Bend on the waist and knees on the equal time as your lower back is right now.

4. Stand without delay up with out compensating for the component with out a weight.

five. Stand right away up.

Precautions: Back want to be straight away and no longer rounded. Select a weight on your competencies if you need to elevate correctly.

Farmers Walk

Movement:

Performed like a stylish deadlift but with 2 bells at your facet. Use heavier weights so the motion is tough. Begin on foot for the prescribed time.

Precautions: Do now not spherical your lower returned and constantly choose a weight you may appropriately flow into.

Hand to Hand Swing

Movement:

1. Begin with everyday swing besides now you will release the bell on the pinnacle of the swing.

2. Grab the bell at the side of your notable hand.

three. Move with a cause.

Precautions: If the bell is simply too an extended way ahead at the same time as you go to take preserve of it allow it move and reset. Choose a weight that you may safely pass.

Hand to Hand Snatch

Movement:

1. Begin the movement with the useful resource of doing the clutch with a swing.

2. Move the bell back off with the equal hand.

 3. Swing the bell once more up and get keep of the bell with the opportunity hand.

4. Move the bell back down and start the transition as required.

Precautions: Ensure you do no longer round your yet again and choose a weight that you can appropriately go with the flow.

Month 1

Day 1

TGU- 3 every aspect alternating

Overhead kb stroll: 30 seconds every facet

KB deadlift 4x5 select out weight, recognition on hinge and lockout

Swing ladders- 3 bells of various sizes, 8 reps each x4

Suitcase deliver- 3 sets of: 30 heavier bell

Single arm deadlift 4x5 every arm

Single arm swings- 4x8 every aspect

Plank 5x: 30

Detailed Explanation:

TGU-three ea. Side alternating. Here you need to reputation on hitting each feature within the flow. Do the left aspect then right component till you do a whole of 6 TGU. Work with a weight you may efficiently cope with. This is not a skip this is achieved rapid, however as an alternative an intentional motion. There not some thing wrong with using even a few thing as moderate as your sneaker for the primary 2 weeks, to learn the movement.

O/H KB Walk 30 seconds every component. Choose your weight carefully right here. You are going to move with the weight overhead for a whole of 30 seconds. Ensure that you lock that arm this is overhead. Walk commonly.

Kettlebell Dead Lift 4 x 5. Choose an appropriate weight, recognition at the hinge and lockout. When it is written 4 x five you'll do four devices of five. There isn't any pre-decided relaxation length right right here. If you pick out a weight that isn't too mild or too heavy, you'll most in all likelihood only need to rest 1 minute.

Swing Ladders-3 bells of various sizes, 8 Reps x four. If you're honestly beginning to apply kettlebells, start moderate. For men a 35# bell is probably the max and girls a 25# bell. Start with the lightest weight do 8 surpassed swings, then circulate to the middle weight and do 8 passed swings, after which bypass to the heaviest weight and do 8 handed swings. You will then relaxation and do it again three extra times.

Suitcase Carry: three devices of 30 seconds. I could use my non-dominate hand first, then dominant, then non-dominate. If you need to rest, absolutely set the load down, rest and resume.

Single Arm Deadlift 4 x 5 every arm. Focus on now not compensating with the arm that is not deciding on the load up. Ensure your decrease once more is immediately. Do 5 reps on one arm, then five reps with the alternative arm. Rest required quantity, and repeat 3 greater instances. Choose a difficult weight right here.

Single Arm Swings 4 x eight every facet. Start with each arm, eight with one arm, 8 with the alternative arm, rest as wanted and do three more times. Ensure you pick a weight you can accurately float.

Plank 5 x :30 seconds. Chances are you received't be able to preserve the plank for 30 seconds. That's properly sufficient, if you could handiest do 10 seconds, relaxation do 10

Day 2

TGU- pause in every position for 5 seconds, 2 every facet

2 hand swings 5x10

Hip flexor stretch

1 hand swing 8L and eight R 6 goblet squats

Repeat 1 hand swings and goblets x4

Hand on hand swings

Do 20 swings, move into: 30 plank repeat x4

Farmers stroll 4 gadgets of: 30 to: forty five seconds

Detailed Explanation:

Turkish Get-Up Pause in ea. Position 5 seconds, 2 ea. Side. Here you can pause on your forearm, palm, knee, and in repute, and do the identical on the way down. Focus on virtually feeling every feature. Ensure you are deciding on a mild weight. There isn't something incorrect with using even some aspect as mild as your sneaker for the number one 2 weeks, to investigate the motion.

2 Hand Swings 5 x 10. You will do 10 repetitions with a weight you may appropriately address. Rest for a brief time, then do this four greater instances.

Hip Flexor Stretch. Really take time to stretch each aspect. Focus on the complete frame here.

1 Hand Swing 8L & 8R/6 Goblet Squats. You will do eight swings collectively together with your left hand, then 8 collectively together with your proper hand, and with same weight flow into proper into doing 6 goblet squats. Rest for loads less than a minute and repeat 3 more times.

Do 20 hand handy swings, then 30 seconds inside the plank. Ensure that you've practiced this motion earlier than doing it for the number one time. If you are doing this in your property, ensure there isn't always some thing that can be broken is inside the manner. If the bell receives far from you, allow it go, and start over. Once you do 20 hand handy swings, you may straight away do 30 seconds in the plank and right away begin with the 20 hand to hand swings. You will do that for an entire of four rounds.

Farmers Walk-four gadgets of 30 seconds to forty five seconds. Choose a heavy enough weight so it is tough, however not so heavy you have to set it down after 15 seconds. Once you hit amongst 30 and forty five seconds, set the burden down, get better, and repeat 3 extra instances.

Day 3

TGU to the popularity characteristic, walk for: 30 seconds then come down, repeat on way down

KB deadlift- 4x5

KB swings 30/30 for 10 mins

Goblet squat 6 reps, at the bottom of the sixth rep curl the kb 6 times with the resource of using the horns, repeat 4 times

30/30 1 arm swings. Swing L then relaxation for: 30, repeat for 8 mins

Hip flexor stretch

Detailed Explanation:

Turkish Get-Up Standing Position Walk 30 seconds then come down, repeat for unique arm. Do a Turkish get-up, then walk for 30 seconds, stop, come down, switch palms, and repeat.

Kettlebell Deadlift 4 x five. Do 5 Repetitions with a weight that isn't slight, but no longer too heavy that you can not entire four devices. Once you do five reps, relaxation for approximately 1 minute, and then do three greater instances. Ensure that your lower back is without delay, and breathe in on the manner down, and out on the way up.

Chapter 5: Living The Healthy Lifestyle

Knowing the way to preserve your purpose weight will assist you keep away from dropping all of your difficult art work as quickly as you have got achieved it. When you attain the point in that you have completed your weight reduction cause, the information you've got got acquired earlier may be useful. You manifestly need to preserve up your newly determined wholesome manner of existence and won't need to break the birthday celebration you may want to have.

Never pass a meal: Keep in mind that your metabolism will interpret this as a sign which you are starving and start to preserve fats as a reserve. Make certain to keep ingesting your food as you've got been making plans them. Furthermore, skipping a meal at one detail in some unspecified time in the future of the day can also additionally moreover bring about overeating in some time even as you're virtually too hungry.

Continue to eat a whole lot of food: This will make it simpler as a way to keep getting all the vitamins and vitamins your body wishes to stay wholesome. It will preserve your frame wholesome, come up with strength, and shield your frame by means of way of doing so. Whole grains, end result, veggies, and lean proteins are a number of the options you've got were given. Keep up your sporting activities! Don't become complacent and prevent walking out right away. If you received education from a private teacher, you presently understand what form of workout is splendid for you and in all likelihood the way to switch subjects up every now and then as nicely.

It's an top notch idea to trade up your routine once in a while to prevent boredom and preserve your body on its ft. You will maintain to stay in shape, experience sturdy and healthy, and you'll further protect your self from illnesses at the same time as you integrate your aerobic and strength education with a wholesome food plan.

Start with in reality 250 extra electricity consistent with day. Check your weight as quickly as every week. Most possibly, you still have a few greater weight to lose. If so, increase your calorie consumption thru some other 250, then weigh yourself every week later.

When you weigh your self at the surrender of the week, maintain going through the ones steps until you be conscious that your weight has stayed the equal. If you've got obtained a touch weight, reduce it thru one hundred calories at a time until it stabilizes and stays the equal from week to week.

Continue ingesting that water: Drink at the least 8 glasses of water each day to preserve your frame functioning properly. Drinking water improves digestion, offers you more electricity, and aids in the natural cleansing of your body. You may even live healthful and hydrated.

Continue to devour often: You have in all likelihood already found out that ingesting 5 to 6 small food an afternoon is a awesome idea because it continues your metabolism going and leaves you feeling glad.

It is vital to hold doing this as well because of the fact, if this grow to be a hassle inside the past, you do now not want to fall into the lure of growing your factor sizes over again. One day you can locate yourself proper lower back in that you began out. You will no a good deal less than located on an entire lot of the weight you worked so difficult to lose all over again.

Keep the junk meals out of doors: Why harm your new healthful conduct via way of reverting to your antique behaviors and overindulging in junk meals? You've found out a manner to meet all of your cravings with scrumptious, nutritious meals. Maintain a each day consumption of fruits and greens of as a minimum six to eight servings.

Take your vitamins every day. Do no longer save you taking your day by day food plan supplements. You can make certain that you get all of the vitamins you want each day through the use of the use of doing this, as a way to additionally assist you hold a healthy weight.

The Secrets of Staying Healthy

Everybody desires to live prolonged and wholesome lives; no character desires to expect getting any excessive ailments. There are techniques to help protect ourselves that can help make our lives extra entire and healthful regular, regardless of the truth that we can't are looking beforehand to or prevent every state of affairs.

You want to prioritize early detection and prevention first. Most humans dread getting their yearly physicals or perhaps going to the dentist every six months for a cleaning. However, retaining those appointments and finding precise scientific doctors will assist you stay healthful because of the reality they could spot matters which you can not.

Knowing your family facts is important because of the truth your medical physician can display your signs and signs and symptoms and carry out routine finding out if there can be a records of maximum cancers or coronary heart sickness in your family.

Respect the corporation you maintain. Spend time with the people who are continuously there for you, collectively along with your companion, children, extended own family, buddies, and coworkers. Enjoy your interactions with others and uphold wholesome friendships. You want those connections on the manner to sense fulfilled in existence.

Sleep for eight hours. Despite the fact that many humans find out this one hard given how busy our lives can become, it's far clearly essential to dwelling a glad and healthy existence.

Find a expertise you excel at. Everybody has moments after they must be doing some thing they in reality experience, and maximum of the time, the ones moments call for their super abilties. Typically, this additionally offers us a first-rate internal feeling and also may be calming and pressure-relieving.

Don't overlook about your pressure; manage it instead! Everyone reviews a few shape of strain, and it is crucial that we manage it to prevent it from turning into overwhelming and taking over our lives.

You can sincerely emerge as bodily sick even as you are plagued thru worry and strain in some of processes. Daily walks will will let you lighten up and take a look at that your time table isn't too complete or which you aren't letting one of a kind human beings's schedules manage your day.

Obtain equilibrium in your life. Try now not to permit artwork devour you or strive no longer to tackle too many projects. Find a balance so you are however able to enjoy all the other subjects spherical you need your pastimes and your buddies and own family.

Even despite the fact that instances can be difficult financially, it's miles nonetheless essential to find time to your family, whom you decide so difficult to guard and offer for.

The Advantages of Staying Healthy

The blessings of preserving appropriate health are limitless. It's now not just that you could in shape into that new outfit and are content material with the way you look. Your average physical, intellectual, and social nicely being are all impacted with the resource of your diploma of health.

Your Physical Health: Maintaining correct bodily health will advantage you in all respects. It now not simplest lets in you to take part in daily sports activities activities like walking, moving, and bending, but it additionally offers you the bodily capacity to appearance after your based circle of relatives contributors.

If you avoid ailments that had been preventable and that could be very high priced, it can be financially immoderate nice.

Your Mental Health: If your mental health is lousy, it's going to moreover have an effect on your physical health. Many humans are blind to the importance in their intellectual fitness to their modern-day day fitness. It should make you sick if you permit your self emerge as overly careworn or if that pressure takes manipulate of your existence.

Your risk of having a coronary heart attack or stroke will increase if you are below strain. You need to find out wholesome techniques to control your pressure, including through exercising, meditation, or remedy. Avoid dealing with pressure in risky techniques, which encompass with the useful useful resource of smoking, ingesting, or eating unhealthful substances.

Disease Prevention: Maintaining ordinary health and staying healthful calls for eating a healthful food regimen. Your health may be right now stricken by the food you select out out to consume.

Phytochemicals are vital for your fitness and might help keep off situations like excessive blood strain, sure styles of maximum cancers, diabetes, and coronary heart ailment. Only positive food, which includes berries, spinach, olives, and kale, incorporate them. Consume a low-fats weight loss program wealthy in whole grains, cease end result, and greens to assist protect your cardiovascular fitness.

Long Life: Maintaining a wholesome manner of life can play a vast feature on your potential to stay an extended and lively existence. Even although you can not prevent all health issues and a number of them are past your control, major a wholesome way of lifestyles can help you avoid the severa maximum essential ones.

Having a wholesome manner of existence that consists of coping with your food regimen is important due to the truth chronic sicknesses like diabetes, coronary coronary heart disorder, maximum cancers, and stroke are the main reasons of lack of existence. Maintaining a healthy weight, how masses you exercise, and the way you control pressure in your existence can all have a vast effect on preventing those ailments.

Maintaining a wholesome way of lifestyles also can increase your spirits, boom your revel in of really worth, and sharpen your mind. You can be extra physically in form, have more patience, and be capable of sleep better at night time.

Improved digestion and reduce blood pressure are more blessings of crucial a wholesome way of life. Maintaining accurate health also let you lessen or absolutely cast off again pain and troubles, in addition to decorate your stability and coordination, posture, and resting heart price.

Chapter 6: Importance Of Strength Training

1.Strength education allows to opposite the lack of muscle mass which decreases with age truely.

2.Increased muscle power improves your posture with upright backbone & facilitates in attaining that "V" fashioned frame.

3.A muscular, leaner & more wholesome frame permits for your notion of "Self-Image" and consequences in better conceitedness & self belief.

four.Strength training allows to increase bone density thereby reducing the threat of osteoporosis & fractures.

5.Strength training allows to maintain joint flexibility and may lessen the symptoms of arthritis.

6.As you benefit muscle, your base metabolic rate has an inclination to growth, due to this making it less tough to govern your weight. This unmarried detail can save you some of ability troubles associated with weight issues & being overweight - first & fundamental of this is Diabetes.

7.Strength education even as paired with cardiovascular schooling allows in strengthening opportunity arterial passages in your coronary coronary heart thereby decreasing blood strain and risk of blocked arteries.

8.Strength training can help alleviate chronic pains like low once more pain & joint pains.

9.Strength education facilitates in reversal in mitochondrial deterioration that commonly happens with growing older.

10.   Strength schooling improves the movement of lymphatic fluid thru your device consequently supporting in green elimination of pollutants.

eleven.   Strength training releases endorphins in mind. Endorphins act as our natural defences within the path of strain and despair. Endorphins are the reason why you experience happy & satisfied after a green session of electricity schooling.

12.   Strength schooling reduces oxidative stress as a end result decreasing risks of most cancers.

thirteen.   Strength education lets you get genuine night time time time sleep therefore having normal first rate effect on your fitness.

Safety Tips for Strength Training

1.Warm up ordinary may be very critical in advance than any energy education regime. It allows to increase blood float to joints and muscle companies, prepares joints for overall overall performance with the aid of manner of enhancing joint mobility, activates your center and hip muscle groups to offer better balance to backbone and hips.

2.Using right shape in the course of electricity education may be very important to lower injuries and maximize income. The carrying activities must be practised with decrease resistance first to master the shape for that routine and then best must you flow into to extended resistance.

3.Working at right tempo allows to maximise the power gains with momentum not interfering with the cause of exercising. Always depend slowly as you carry out the exercising, therefore controlling motion and offer a slight pause in among as you attain at maximum resistance effect. Do not permit the momentum of the motion preserve on till the prevent. Never lose manipulate of the motion.

four.Keep breathing slowly and never hold your breath within the course of exercise to avoid assemble-up of your blood pressure. Generally, you need to exhale as you figure against resistance & inhale as you release.

five.Keep tough the muscles thru the use of slowly increasing the resistance. The preference of resistance want to be such that on the surrender of 1 set of repetition the focused muscle or agency of muscle groups have to be worn-out (however no longer too tired) and the workout can despite the fact that be finished in right form. When you revel in the resistance turning into less complex, upload more resistance or upload a hard and fast.

6.Ideally you want to exercising all essential muscle groups of your frame 2-three times every week. This can be done thru dividing regimes into pinnacle and reduce body muscle mass additives and doing them on separate days, repeating each trouble at the least 2-3 instances in step with week or doing whole frame sports activities 2-three times per week.

7.Tiny tears upward thrust up in muscle groups because of electricity schooling which need to be healed. These tears make the muscles increase stronger after re-modelling. At least forty eight hours need to accept to each muscle to get higher before similarly strength education.

8.Cut again on the exercising (lessen resistance or reduce the devices) if you revel in large ache, dizziness, breathlessness at some degree within the consultation or sense tired at a few degree within the day.

nine.Always preserve a moderate bend in knees and elbows at the identical time as straightening legs and arms all through physical sports. Locking the ones joints at the acute ends of your resistance workout can motive accidents.

10. Cool down with entire body stretches after the consultation. Five-10 mins settle down sports activities should be right.

Chapter 7: Why Exercise With Kettlebells

Kettlebell carrying occasions are an effective & much less highly-priced way of doing muscle strengthening and cardiovascular workout. It's a excellent device to do whole frame exercise as you could art work many muscle companies with a single kettlebell.

The gadget is easy to move and may be stored in a small vicinity. You do now not constantly want an complicated gym setup to do the carrying occasions. It can without troubles be finished at domestic or your place of job.

In this ebook, via little by little commands, I will manual you to the constant and effective techniques of the use of Kettlebells for Strength Training. Emphasis may be laid on the right greedy of the kettlebell, right begin characteristic and accurate movement of the specific frame detail for the popular consequences.

Why to Choose the Correct Kettlebell Weight

Choosing the right kettlebell weight can be very vital to get the desired consequences from the bodily activities. Less kettlebell weight may additionally moreover furthermore reason vain consequences inside the direction of muscle strengthening, staying energy and lots of others. On the other aspect a very heavy kettlebell can purpose muscle traces and joint injuries.

How to Choose the Correct Kettlebell Weight

To apprehend a manner to pick out the kettlebell weight we first want to apprehend how wearing activities are finished. Kettlebell sporting sports activities are completed as units of repetitions. A repetition is completing one exercising and a difficult and rapid is a collection of repetitions.

The choice of a particular kettlebell weight is based upon on how without problem you can complete a set of 8-10 repetitions with the chosen weight. With the best weight you need to be able to do 8-10 repetitions without trouble (however not too outcomes furthermore). At the end of the set your muscle tissue start feeling tired and you may struggle a piece to complete the set.

You could make out if the kettlebell is sincerely too heavy even as you begin straining your lower back or swinging your body to elevate the load or perform the workout.

Important Tips for Kettlebell Exercise Program

• If you're new to kettlebell, start slowly. It is critical to analyze the right shape and technique of the exercise. Follow the little by little instructions stated on this ebook to get the correct exercising form.

• Kettlebell has a bent to swing. Practice managing it first, get used to the texture and motion of the kettlebell in hands earlier than you operate it for exercising.

• Learn the method and shape of the workout with the lighter weight first. Once you're comfortable, flow into to heavier weights or greater reps and units.

• Complete the regime at least instances every week to get suitable results. Any range less than that won't be useful and you may experience demotivated to maintain.

• Once you're cushty with the carrying occasions (this is, you have got had been given constructed up enough stamina and power), repeat the classes three-four times in keeping with week.

• Be organized to feel little sore in muscle mass and moreover occasionally joints as you start with the exercise application. This is regular and might subside in an afternoon or . As you preserve with the training the bodily sports activities will become less tough and additional cushty. However, if you enjoy a shocking or sharp pain at some stage in or after the exercising, proper now prevent doing the workout.

• Rest for an afternoon some of the classes. Once you've constructed up the stamina and strength you may do 3-four periods every week.

• Try switching kettlebell exercising with cardiovascular education. Going for walks on change days with kettlebell workout enables to collect your stamina. Even with this, take 1-2 days of relaxation in every week. Do not overstrain.

• Reduce quantity of gadgets but carry out all of the sports, in case you experience an excessive amount of strained with the regime. In case of any scientific motive to prevent a selected exercise, replace the workout with some different exercising.

• Ensure right hydration. Do not allow yourself get dehydrated within the direction of workout. Replenish any lack of water through sweat with water or electrolytes.

• Wear suitable shoes while workout in particular if you are diabetic, have flat foot or have pronated foot.

Kettlebell Holding Positions

The kettlebell, in evaluation to dumbbell, is a really numerous training device which can be held in a number of strategies. As the kettlebell weight is offset from the address, the cease end result you purchased range with the region in which you hold the kettlebell.

Here are unique positions in which kettlebell may be held in conjunction with their benefits and downsides.

1.Two handed maintain

This is one of the simple and most effective positions used in kettlebell maintaining.

Hold the kettlebell manipulate with every arms in the overhand grip. Use the proper form of kettlebell for this function. Some kettlebells are designed most effective for one hand and so using this defensive function may be very tough and can experience cramped.

Typical bodily activities finished with this function: Kettlebell Slingshot, Kettlebell Good Morning, Swing variations & Romanian

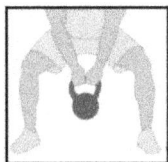

Deadlift

2.Single exceeded maintain via the use of the use of the body

This is one of the maximum well-known keeping role in kettlebell physical games. It locations extra load on shoulder and creates a rotational stress on frame which wants to be counterbalanced with the aid of the use of center muscle companies. Since it places greater stress on grip and forearm muscle tissues, novices find it tough.

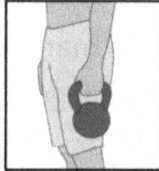

Typical sporting sports activities done with this feature: Biceps Curls, Kettlebell Rows, Single Arm Swings, Single Arm / Leg Deadlift versions & Kettlebell High Pulls.

three.By the body maintain

This is the very nice way to keep the kettlebell. A style of sports activities may be performed on this function in a consistent and controlled manner.

The kettlebell is held with the thumbs throughout the deal with and the relaxation of the hands maintain the frame of the kettlebell. The kettlebell is held near the

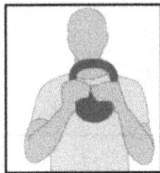

chest.

However, a few humans favor to maintain the kettlebell by way of way of using the horns.

Irrespective of the shape of 'By the body maintain' used by you, it want to no longer make any realistic difference to the mechanics of the sports activities activities completed with this retaining position. Although, you may need to readjust the kettlebell function on occasion as it has a dishonest to slip after a few actions.

Typical sporting sports activities carried out with this feature: Squats, Lunges, Staggered Stance Triceps Press & Kettlebell Bob and Weave.

4.Goblet preserve

It is a cushty manner of retaining the kettlebell.

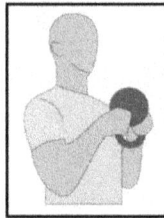

The kettlebell is held with each arms on the horns, with the body of kettlebell up. This characteristic places more call for on wrist muscle organizations due to the fact the goblet can flip and flop backwards and forwards. To counteract the instability, you may relaxation the goblet against the chest because the fatigue units in.

Typical physical video video games completed with this function: Kettlebell Halo & its variations.

5.Rack keep

This preserve is essential to comprehend as you make stronger in kettlebell schooling.

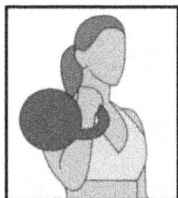

Kettlebell is held without problems towards the aspect of the shoulder, at the outer trouble of the forearm, with the arm tucked in, wrist right away, shoulder down and Latissimus Dorsi muscle engaged.

When engaged nicely, you can maintain it for prolonged time frame without getting fatigued. However in case you wing out the elbow and maintain kettlebell out and not near shoulder, the region will cause fatigue very quickly.

Typical physical video video games achieved with this feature: Clean, Overhead Press, Squat and Lunge variations.

6.Overhead maintain

This hold is important to recognize as you

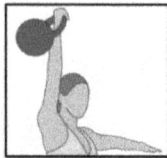

boom in kettlebell schooling.

In the overhead kettlebell role, the kettlebell is held in underhand grip with the body of the kettlebell resting in competition to the wrist / forearm and the wrist locked first-rate and at once to protect it.

The kettlebell used for underhand kettlebell function have to be nicely designed. A badly designed kettlebell can pinch the wrist or experience very uncomfortable in the direction of the forearm.

Typical bodily video video games accomplished with this characteristic: Turkish

Get-Up, Windmill, Overhead Press and Snatch & Overhead Squats.

7.Bottoms up maintain

This is the most hard of the kettlebell maintaining positions requiring brilliant alignment at some stage inside the arm and body similarly to wrist energy and balance.

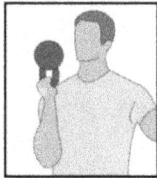

The kettlebell is held firmly in the underhand grip with address down and body up, maintaining the wrist straight away.

Be cautious and stay in a characteristic to be able to get out of the manner or perhaps drop the kettlebell if crucial.

Typical wearing activities completed with this function: Bottom-Up Clean

Chapter 8: Warm-Up Exercises

To stay safe and prepare your frame for wearing activities you have to constantly do a little warmth americabefore the electricity sporting occasions. The warm up physical video video games assist to growth the temperature and unfasten the muscle corporations in advance than the heavy body muscle paintings. Warm u.S.Improve the body

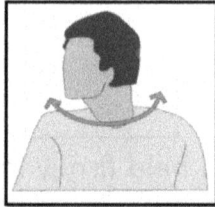

usual ordinary overall performance and save you accidents. These bodily sports activities want to be dynamic carrying sports like skipping, running at a place, chest expansion & rotations. About 5 mins' heat united states of america of americaare sufficient to make your cardiovascular device organized.

The following warm up physical games are top notch to prepare your frame for an excessive workout.

1. Neck Rotations:

Stand tall along side your chin parallel to the floor. Exhale and take your chin to the chest. Inhale, rotate your neck and take your chin toward the left shoulder (look over your left shoulder). Exhale and get your chin decrease returned to the chest feature. Inhale, rotate your neck and take your chin to the proper shoulder (appearance over your proper shoulder). Get your chin all over again to the chest feature as you exhale. Move you chin as a exceptional deal due to the fact the begin feature as you inhale. Repeat three times.

2. Shoulder Backward Rotations:

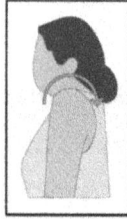

Stand tall with chin parallel to the ground and shoulders handling ahead. Take your shoulders beforehand. Start rotating the shoulders taking them up and in the back of. Get your shoulder-blades collectively as you move the shoulders in the back of. Get shoulders once more to the begin function.

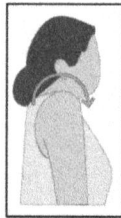

three. Shoulder Forward Rotations:

Stand tall with chin parallel to the floor and shoulders handling forward. Take your shoulders in the back of, getting your shoulder blades collectively. Continue rotating the shoulders taking them up and forwards. Get shoulders again to the start feature. Repeat this collection 10 instances.

4. Chest Expansions:

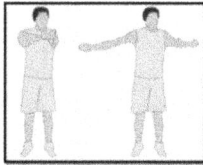

Stand tall with chin parallel to the floor and shoulders going via in advance. Raise your arms to the shoulder degree and take them lower back setting up the chest. Repeat 10 instances.

five. Torso Rotations:

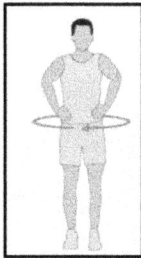

Stand tall with feet hip width distance apart. Place your fingers on the waist and rotate your trunk clockwise. Repeat 10 times. Then rotate your trunk anti-clockwise. Repeat 10 instances.

6. Arm Rotations:

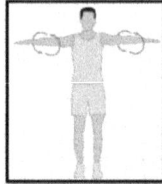

Stand tall along with your ft hip width distance aside. Raise your palms to the aspect at shoulder degree. Make circles with your fingers transferring them clockwise and anti-clockwise (10 times in every course).

7. Side Arm Raises:

Stand tall at the side of your toes hip width distance aside. Raise your every palms sideways up 10 times.

eight. Sideward Bending:

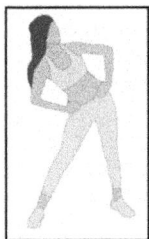

Stand tall together along with your toes greater than hip width distance aside, hands positioned at the waist. Start bending aspect to side. Repeat it 10 times.

nine. Torso Swings:

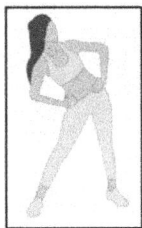

Stand tall with ft greater than hip width distance apart. Bend in advance at the waist with hands stretched to the rims. Start swinging on the torso conducting contrary

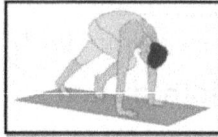

hand to the foot. Repeat alternately on each factors, 10 times

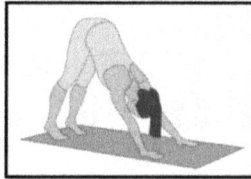

10. Lunge:

A. Come in a downward canine pose.

B. Take your proper knee toward nose and step your proper foot between arms to come in a lunge. The knee perspective need to now not skip underneath 900 regardless of the reality that.

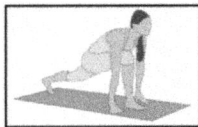

C. Reverse the movement and repeat on the opposite component.

11. Hip Rotation

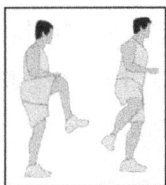

Lift your right leg and balance your body at the left foot. Rotate your leg at the hips in clockwise path 10 times. Next rotate it in contrary direction 10 times. Repeat with the alternative leg.

12. Jog on Spot

Jog immediately. Try to elevate your legs excessive enough to make your thighs parallel to the floor. Do 20 jogs of each foot.

13. Side to Side Hop

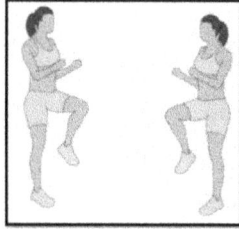

Balance yourself on one foot with the opportunity leg raised excessive. Hop on the raised leg facet, bringing that one down and raising the opportunity leg up simultaneously. Repeat this 20 times.

14. Kettlebell Halo

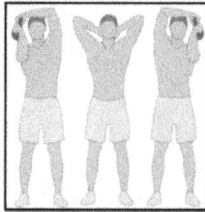

Stand tall with ft shoulder width aside, and hold the kettlebell in goblet role in the front of your chest. Raise the left elbow up as you are taking the kettlebell in the lower back of your head, rotate throughout the pinnacle after which drift it the front as you get right elbow up. Bring the kettlebell once more to front. Repeat it 10 times. Repeat 10 times in contrary path. Do no longer permit kettlebell to move too an extended manner a long way from head in some unspecified time in the future of movement. Stabilise the hips and save you it from transferring. Keep your middle engaged by means of using tucking in stomach at a few stage inside the movement.

15. Kettlebell Slingshot

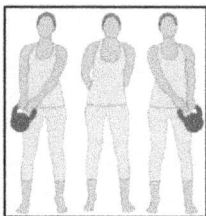

Stand tall with toes shoulder width apart and keep the kettlebell in hand grip with fingers right away. Rotate the Kettlebell across the body in a round motion for the duration of the hips. Change the grip to 1 hand maintain thru letting skip of 1 hand as you are taking the kettlebell within the again of your frame. Pass the kettlebell from one hand to the alternative right now inside the again of the hips. Change the grip to two hand maintain as

129

you bring the kettlebell lower back to the the the front from the alternative thing. Rotate it 10 instances clockwise and 10 times anti clockwise. Keep the kettlebell close to the body. Keep the shoulders down at some stage in the movement. Stabilise your hips as you rotate the kettlebell.

16. Kettlebell Good Morning

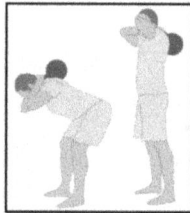

Stand tall together together together with your ft shoulder width apart and preserve the kettlebell within the goblet function, in the back of your top lower returned. Taking weight thru the heels and maintaining knees smooth, hinge ahead at your waist, pushing the buttocks backwards. Reverse the movement and are available lower returned to the upright feature. Repeat it 10 instances. Ensure that the neck stays regular with the lower lower returned throughout the movement. Bend from the hips and no longer from decrease lower back through pushing buttocks backwards. Keep the elbows close to collectively as you do the exercise. At the pinnacle of the motion squeeze the buttocks tight. Don't lock the knees. Keep them soft at some point of the movement.

Warm-up Sets: Every exercising session want initially a heat up set. Warm up set consists of all the sports activities activities you can do, at the aspect of your smallest or no kettlebell for 10-15 repetitions with slower than everyday pace.

Chapter 9: Upper Body Exercises

Biceps & Forearm Exercises

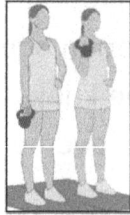

Biceps Curl

Effect:Strengthens the biceps muscle tissues.

Difficulty Level: Beginner

Start Position: Stand tall collectively together with your ft hip width distance apart, keeping kettlebell in unmarried hand role with underhand grip, with the beneficial useful resource of the factor of your frame.

Steps:

1.Bend your arm at elbow taking the kettlebell as lots due to the fact the shoulder with out transferring the higher arm.

2.Hold the kettlebell up for one second.

three.Slowly get the kettlebell all of the manner down to the start characteristic.

four.Repeat it 10 times.

five.Repeat 10 times with the opportunity arm.

Fine Tips:

1.Keep the elbow tucked to the facet of the torso as you do the motion.

2.Engage biceps muscle as you do the motion.

three.Avoid swaying of shoulder throughout movement to prevent giving momentum to the movement.

Kettlebell Row

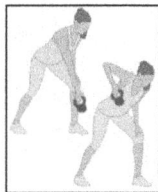

Effect:Strengthens all over again, biceps and shoulder muscle groups. Improves stability of center and decrease once more.

Difficulty Level: Beginner

Start Position: Stand in a staggered stance along side your knees barely bent, keeping a kettlebell in single hand function with overhand grip, definitely above your the front foot for your contrary arm. Lean in advance collectively collectively together with your lower again directly and head up. Rest your unfastened arm in your the front leg for balance.

Steps:

1.Pull the kettlebell as heaps because the side of the torso retaining the elbow tucked through the use of the element.

2.Pause on the pinnacle feature for a 2d.

3.Slowly lower down the kettlebell to the begin role.

four.Repeat it 10 times.

Fine Tips:

1.Do no longer allow the shoulder slouch and maintain the shoulder blades lower back on the pinnacle of the row.

2.Maintain the posture alignment finally of the movement. Do no longer permit the decrease again curve every time during the movement.

3.Pull the kettlebell as a good deal because the rib level.

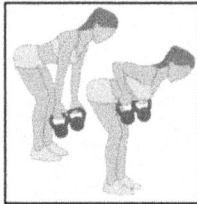

Double Kettlebell Row

Effect:Strengthens again, biceps and shoulder muscle companies. Improves stability of center and lower once more.

Difficulty Level: Beginner

Start Position: Stand with toes hip width distance aside, preserving your weight on the heels and knees barely bent. Hold a kettlebell in each hands, in unmarried handed preserve with the useful resource of the rims of your frame and bend your torso at hips to forty five levels in order that the kettlebells preserve near at the shin degree on each facets.

Steps:

1.Row every the kettlebells up closer to the hips, pulling with the aid of your elbows.

2.Pause on the top for two seconds and squeeze your shoulder blades.

three.Reverse the movement and get the kettlebell to the begin characteristic.

4.Repeat it 6-eight times.

Fine Tips:

1.Keep your over again flat from shoulders to hips during the motion.

2.The rowing pull need to go back from elbows and not from neck or better again.

Keep your shoulders pulled within the course of the hips all through the movement.

three.The movement must be sluggish and controlled.

4.Pull and decrease the kettlebell on the same time, keeping the symmetry.

Triceps Exercises

Staggered Stance Triceps Press

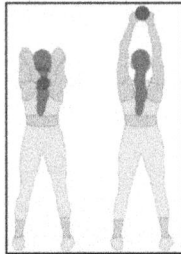

Effect:This exercising strengthens the triceps and shoulder muscular tissues.

Difficulty Level: Beginner

Start Position: Stand tall inside the staggered stance. Hold a kettlebell via the horns with each arms, in the back of your pinnacle returned, with elbows up and arms via the side of your head.

Steps:

1.Raise the kettlebell overhead, straightening your elbows, maintaining the palms with the beneficial resource of the component of your head.

2.Slowly decrease the kettlebell to the begin position, maintaining the elbows tucked through the issue of your head.

3.Repeat it 10 instances.

Fine Tips:

1.The motion have to be slow and controlled.

2.Keep your chest up and decrease returned tall in some unspecified time in the future of the movement.

Bottom Up Clean

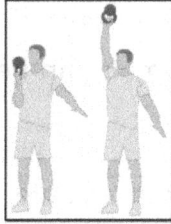

Effect:This exercise strengthens the shoulder stabilizer muscular tissues. It improves shoulder mobility and center stability.

Difficulty Level: Advanced

Start Position: Stand tall with ft extra than shoulder width apart. Hold the kettlebell in backside up function with wrist instantly, elbow bent and tucked through the issue of your body.

Steps:

1.Press the kettlebell overhead, closer to the ceiling, preserving the wrist straight away.

2.Slowly decrease the kettlebell down.

three.Repeat it 10 times.

4.Repeat 10 times on the other side.

Fine Tips:

1.Static exercise preserve: Start with 5 2d bottoms up easy maintain before progressing to overhead keep.

2.Maintain an remarkable alignment with again tall and kettlebell in line of straight wrist, proper now elbow and shoulder inside the overhead feature.

3.Hold the kettlebell with a company grip ensuring that the kettlebell does no longer flop again over and hit you. Always be in a place wherein you could speedy step apart out of the way of kettlebell in case it falls.

Shoulder Exercises

Kettlebell Swing

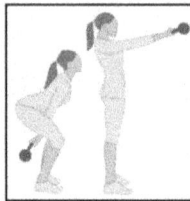

Effect:Strengthens core, lower frame and shoulders. Improves strength for your hips.

Difficulty Level: Beginner

Start Position: Stand tall together with your feet hip width distance aside, protecting kettlebell in passed keep with an overhand grip within the the front of your thighs.

Steps:

1.Lower your hip down and decrease lower again as you hinge your torso on the hips, bringing the torso parallel to the ground and taking the kettlebell between your legs with arms at once.

2.With a thrust, push the hips earlier, swinging the kettlebell beforehand and upward until the kettlebell reaches the shoulder diploma.

three.Bring the kettlebell down and move returned to the start characteristic.

four.Repeat the gathering 10 instances.

Fine Tips:

1.Do now not depend on the arm muscle tissue to swing the kettlebell. The swinging momentum need to be generated with the aid of manner of using in advance thrust on the hips.

2.Completely end the rep and squeeze your glutes on the top.

One Arm Swing

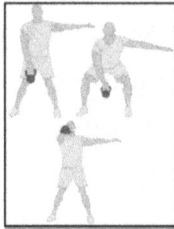

Effect:Improves cardiovascular patience. Strengthens the glutes, hamstrings and hip flexors. Improves shoulder muscle groups energy and mobility.

Difficulty Level: Intermediate

Start Position: Stand tall with feet extra than hip width distance apart, ft pointing outwards at 20 levels. Hold the kettlebell in a single hand in overhand grip inside the front of your thigh. The different arm is prolonged to the facet, parallel to the floor.

Steps:

1.Bring the hips down and once more and bend at waist, swinging the kettlebell among your thighs. Keep your chest in advance, again right away and middle engaged as you try this motion.

2.Thrust your hips forward as you squeeze the glutes, swinging kettlebell forward and upward till the shoulder level.

3.Return the kettlebell to the start function.

four.Repeat it 10 times.

five.Repeat with the alternative arm.

Fine Tips:

1.Keep your center engaged and chest ahead at a few stage within the motion.

2.The swinging motion of the arm comes from the thrust generated at hips, without counting on the arm muscle agencies.

Step Out Swing

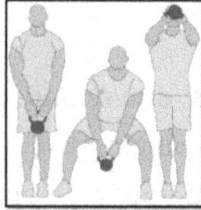

Effect:Strengthens the leg muscle corporations, specially hamstrings, glutes and quadriceps. Improves core stability. Strengthens shoulder muscle tissues.

Difficulty Level: Beginner

Start Position: Stand tall with ft together, preserving one kettlebell with every hands in an overhand grip in front of your thighs.

Steps:

1.Step to a factor with one foot, bringing your hips down and lower back, taking the kettlebell returned, amongst your legs.

2.Step lower back to the begin characteristic as you thrust the hips forward, swinging the kettlebell as much as the shoulder diploma after which bringing it lower lower back within the front of the thighs.

3.Repeat it 10 times.

Fine Tips:

1.As you swing the kettlebell between your legs, enjoy the tension in glutes and hamstrings.

2.The upward swinging motion of the kettlebell comes from the thrust generated at hips, without counting on arm muscular tissues engagement.

3.Keep your center engaged and do now not arch your decrease lower back as you do the motion.

Staggered Stance Halo

Effect:This workout strengthens shoulders, fingers, middle muscle tissue. It improves shoulder mobility and frame stability.

Difficulty Level: Intermediate

Start Position: Hold the horns of the kettlebell with the bell coping with up at chest peak.

Steps:

1.Take a huge bounce forward together with your right foot so your toes are staggered. Keep your knees gentle (no longer locked).

2.Lift the bell and slowly circle it round your head in a clockwise path.

three.Return to the start function; then circle the kettlebell spherical your head in anti-clockwise direction.

4.Return to starting characteristic. Both clockwise & anticlockwise motion equals 1 repetition. Do eight-10 reps, then repeat with the alternative leg staggered in advance.

Fine Tips:

1.Do not permit kettlebell to transport too some distance a ways from head throughout motion.

2.Stabilise the hips and hold them squared because of this stopping them from transferring.

3.Keep your middle engaged through tucking in abdomen at some point of the motion.

Overhead Hold & Walk

Effect:This workout strengthens shoulder stabilizer muscle agencies. It improves middle electricity and balance.

Difficulty Level: Beginner

Start Position: Stand tall with feet shoulder width aside and preserve a kettlebell overhead inside the proper hand with wrist at once, elbow locked, shoulders lower lower back and down within the socket.

Steps:

1.Start on foot tall with the kettlebell inside the overhead characteristic.

2.Walk for 60 seconds.

3.Walk with the kettlebell held overhead in left hand for 60 seconds.

4.Repeat twice on every components.

Fine Tips:

1.Keep the frame tall and middle engaged in the route of the movement.

2.Choose the kettlebell weight which you may preserve statically overhead for 30 seconds, earlier than walking with it.

3.Keep the overhead arm strong on the identical time as walking.

4.This exercising can be made challenging with the resource of maintaining kettlebells in every arms in overhead maintain.

Chest Exercises

Kettlebell Fly

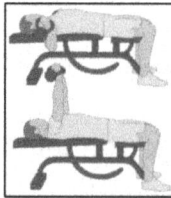

Effect:This exercising Improves the strength of hands and chest muscle corporations.

Difficulty Level: Beginner

Start Position: Lie down right away at the bench protecting kettlebell in every hand with underhand grip, arms kidnapped and elbows bent at ninety degrees. The legs are bent at knees at 90 levels with feet supported on the floor, hip width distance apart.

Steps:

1.Push the kettlebell instantly up, extending your palms.

2.Hold it inside the up function for 1 second.

three.Slowly reverse the movement reducing kettlebell all of the manner all the way down to the start function.

Chapter 10: Lower Body Exercises

Quadriceps Exercises

Kettlebell Squat

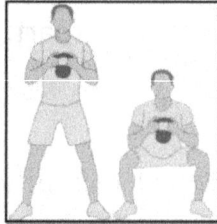

Effect: This workout strengthens the muscle mass of decrease frame and improves middle stability.

Difficulty Level: Beginner

Start Position: Stand tall with toes shoulder width aside. Hold a kettlebell with each palms via the horns, in front of the chest, close to the body.

Steps:

1.Lower your frame down right into a squat, through the use of pushing the hips lower back and down, till your thighs are parallel to the floor. Keep the kettlebell near the chest.

2.Reverse the motion and go back to the start function.

three.Repeat it 10 times.

Fine Tips

1.Do now not permit the knees cave inward or flow the ft in the front.

2.Keep your torso tall and chest forward within the route of the movement.

Static Lunge & Press

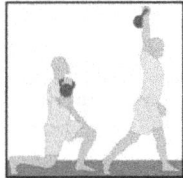

Effect: This exercising strengthens middle, glutes, hamstrings, quadriceps, shoulder and decrease returned muscle companies. It improves center stability and body balance. It improves cardiovascular staying power.

Difficulty Level: Intermediate

Start Position:Stand tall with ft shoulder width apart and preserve kettlebell in rack feature within the proper hand. Get proper into a lunge, sliding proper foot at once inside the back of.

Steps:

1.Raise your body up via pushing into the left foot, straightening the left leg. Both toes live on the begin function as you do the motion.

2.Press the kettlebell right away up from the rack function, as you come inside the up function.

three.Reverse the movement and go back to the start role.

4.Repeat the gathering 10 instances.

five.Repeat 10 instances on the other thing.

Fine Tips:

1.Keep your middle engaged at some stage inside the motion.

2.Keep your toes planted as you do the motion.

three.Keep the hips and shoulders squared at a few level in the motion.

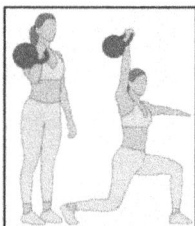

Reverse Lunge with Kettlebell Press

Effect: This exercising strengthens center, legs and shoulder muscle tissue. It improves balance of middle and lower frame. It improves shoulder and legs mobility.

Difficulty Level: Intermediate

Start Position: Stand tall with ft hip width distance aside and center engaged. Hold the kettlebell in your proper hand in a racked role at shoulder top with palm going thru in and the kettlebell resting at the outer thing of proper forearm.

153

Steps:

1.Step returned on the aspect of your proper foot and bend every knees to 90 levels to drop proper right into a lunge.

2.As you drop into the lunge, press the kettlebell straight away up extending your hand overhead. You may additionally expand your left arm to the issue to help with balance.

three.Push off into the right foot to get lower back to the begin feature. Lower the kettlebell proper all the way all the way down to the rack function.

4.Repeat above collection 10 instances.

5.Repeat it 10 times at the left aspect.

Fine Tips:

1.Keep your middle engaged and torso tall at some point of the movement.

2.Do not allow the knees fall down or permit the the the front knee pass the toes ahead during the movement.

3.Keep the hips and shoulders squared (going thru ahead) and do now not lean to at least one facet or flip the torso as you do the motion.

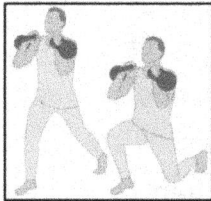

Racked Split Squat Lunge

Effect: This exercising strengthens the middle, glutes, quadriceps and hamstrings. It works on frame balance. Staying within the break up stance maintains your leg muscle tissues engaged at some stage in the exercise as a result improving body endurance.

Difficulty Level: Intermediate

Start Position: Hold a kettlebell in each hand in the racked function in order that your hands are handling every different and the bells are striking down and resting for your shoulders. Stand tall collectively along side your toes shoulder-width aside. Step forward about 2 toes collectively along with your proper foot and plant it firmly on the floor.

Steps:

1.Bend each knees to ninety tiers and drop right right into a lunge. Your proper quad and left shin need to be about parallel to the ground. Your torso want to be tall with again flat and not arched or rounded. Your proper knee must be above your proper foot. Keep your hips and core engaged.

2.Push via the heel of your proper foot to move lower again to the begin feature.

3.Do 10 repetitions.

4.Then do 10 repetitions with the left foot ahead.

Fine Tips:

1.Keep your center engaged in some unspecified time in the future of the movement.

2.Keep the hips and shoulders squared (going through beforehand) and do now not flip the torso as you do the movement.

3.Do now not allow your knees to provide way all through the motion.

four.Do no longer allow your the the front knee pass the ft earlier.

Bulgarian Lunge

Effect: This is an effective preparatory exercise for single leg kettlebell physical video video games. It strengthens middle, quadriceps, hamstrings and glutes. It improves frame stability.

Difficulty Level: Intermediate

Start Position: Stand tall in step fame with the rear foot placed on a step. The distance some of the ft must be extensive sufficient to do a deep lunge. Hold the kettlebell with each arms close to chest in the the front of the body.

Steps:

1.Drop proper right into a lunge, getting the the the front thigh parallel to the floor.

2.Push all over again to the start characteristic.

three.Repeat it 10 times.

four.Repeat 10 times on the opposite aspect.

Fine Tips:

1.Keep your center engaged and chest up within the direction of the motion.

2.Beginners can begin with the low step.

3.If you suffer from toe problems, you may located instep on the stepper simply so foot is flat on the stepper.

4.Keep your hips and shoulders squared (going through in advance) in the path of the movement.

five.Do no longer allow your knee give manner or bypass the toes within the the front on the identical time as in the lunge.

Hamstring Exercises

Romanian Deadlift

Effect: This workout strengthens decrease

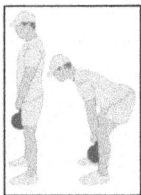

lower again, glutes and hamstring muscle groups.

Difficulty Level: Beginner

Start Position: Stand tall with ft shoulder width apart, keeping one kettlebell bell with both fingers in overhand grip, in front of your thighs.

Steps:

1.Hinge your torso forwards at your hips, as you are taking the hips returned, retaining the palms instantly and kettle bell close to the body. Slightly bend your knees as you do the movement.

2.Reverse the movement enticing your center and pass returned to the begin feature. Squeeze your glutes as you attain to the start feature, preserving the backbone impartial.

three.Repeat the movement 10 times.

Fine Tips

1.Keep the shoulder down and once more and do not spherical your another time for the duration of the motion. Keep the neck unbiased at a few degree within the motion.

2.Keep the kettlebell close to your body during the motion.

three.Do no longer over reap down and lock the knees.

Glutes Exercises

Kettlebell Leg Raises

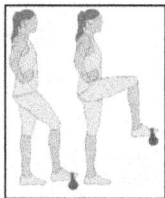

Effect: This exercise strengthens hip and knee flexors, stomach and reduce another time muscle tissues. Improves middle balance.

Difficulty Level: Intermediate

Start Position: Stand tall with ft shoulder width aside and arms resting at the waist. Hook a kettlebell at the foot and curl the ft in the direction of your body.

Steps:

1.Bend the leg with the kettlebell until your hip and knee come at ninety stages.

2.Pause and reduce the leg down.

three.Repeat it 10 times.

4.Repeat 10 instances on the opposite side.

Fine Tips

1.Maintain tall and upright characteristic throughout the motion.

Single Leg Deadlift

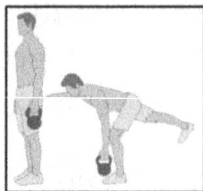

Effect: This workout strengthens hips, decrease lower back and middle muscles. It develops a sturdy connection among top and decrease frame through bypass body middle muscle tissue. It improves frame stability.

Difficulty Level: Advanced

Start Position: Stand tall preserving kettlebell in left hand.

Steps:

1.Standing on the left leg, pivot your frame on the hip, taking it down, preserving the once more and right leg within the right now line. Do now not allow the kettlebell to drag the shoulder down. Keep the shoulder again in its socket.

2.Reverse the motion and skip lower back to the begin characteristic.

three.Repeat it 10 times.

four.Repeat 10 times at the alternative aspect.

Fine Tips

1.Do now not allow the rear leg to rotate outwards, interest on pointing your ft in the direction of the ground.

2.The movement need to be slow and controlled.

three.Engage your center and hip muscular tissues as you do the movement.

Chapter 11: Core Exercises

Kettlebell Sit-up

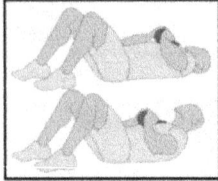

Effect: This is a center strengthening exercise which enables to enhance belly muscle tissues, lower once more muscle mass and hip flexors. Improves stability of middle.

Difficulty Level: Beginner

Start Position: Lie down right away for your decrease returned with knees bent at ninety stages and feet flat at the floor. Hold the kettlebell in every hands, on top of the chest.

Steps:

1.Imprint your lower back, attractive the center. Keeping the kettlebell in opposition on your chest, raise your torso, doing a crunch with the aid of manner of contracting belly muscle corporations.

2.Pause at the top for a second.

3.Slowly decrease the torso again to the ground retaining the middle engaged.

4.Repeat it 10 instances.

Fine Tips:

1.Keep your center engaged at some diploma inside the movement.

2.The movement want to be slow and managed.

three.Do now not tuck your chin too much, use your stomach muscular tissues to do the crunch.

Kettlebell High Pulls

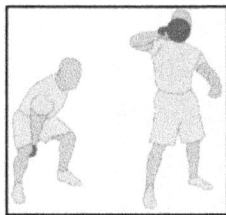

Effect: This exercising improves energy and balance of complete frame. It improves cardiovascular staying power. It strengthens center, buttocks, hamstrings, decrease again, shoulders, triceps and pinnacle lower back muscle agencies.

Difficulty Level: Intermediate

Start Position: Stand in a partial squat function collectively with your ft little wider than shoulder width apart. Hold the kettlebell in the right hand, the various legs, inside the overhand grip with arm at once. Extend the left arm at the back of.

Steps:

1.Thrust your body up, coming to the popularity feature as you swing the kettlebell as much as the shoulder degree. Row yet again the kettlebell at this horizontal function preserving forearm in line with kettlebell with wrist tight. Bring the left arm beforehand to maintain the steadiness.

2.Pause at the top for a second and squeeze your shoulder blade muscle tissues.

3.Reverse the motion and move returned to the begin function.

four.Repeat the sequence 10 instances.

Fine Tips:

1.Control the kettlebell just so it does not slam your arm subsequently of the motion.

2.Use elbow to row the kettlebell.

Overhead Straight Arm Sit-up

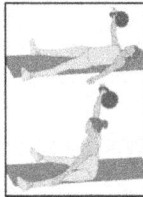

Effect:This workout strengthens the shoulder stabilizer muscle groups. It improves core power.

Difficulty Level: Advanced

Start Position: Lie down right now in your again with legs hip width distance apart. Hold the kettlebell inside the proper hand with arm vertical to the floor, wrist instantly and elbow locked.

Steps:

1.Engage your center and get to the sitting function as you circulate the kettlebell up and press it up closer to the ceiling.

2.Reverse the motion and are available to the begin function.

3.Repeat it 10 times.

four.Repeat 10 times at the left side.

Fine Tips:

1.Imprint your lower lower again to have interaction the core after which come to sitting feature, keeping the core engaged within the route of the movement.

2.Keep your legs right now and arm locked out straight away as you sit up.

three.If your hamstrings are tight your knees may additionally additionally barely bend as you sit up.

four.You may also additionally moreover barely perspective the kettlebell beforehand from vertical to help in starting off the sit up.

five.At the top of the exercising supply the chest up and preserve the shoulders once more and down.

6.Lower from top characteristic to floor in a slow and controlled manner, resisting the pull of gravity.

"The fight is obtained or lost a long way away from witnesses, in the lower back of the strains, inside the health club, and accessible on the road, prolonged in advance than I dance below those lighting."

– Muhammad Ali

Chapter 12: Full Body Exercises

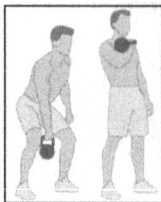

Kettlebell Clean

Effect: This exercising activates entire body. It strengthens middle, hips, hamstrings, quadriceps, again stabilizers, deltoids, trapezius and shoulder stabilizers. It enables to develop sturdy and explosive hips for sports activities. It additionally improves cardiovascular staying energy.

Difficulty Level: Beginner

Start Position: Stand tall with toes shoulder width apart and location the kettlebell in the front of your ft.

Steps:

1.Lift the kettlebell in unmarried hand function, thru snapping the hips in advance and take it as masses as the chest, as if zipping the jacket. Wrap your arm at some point of the kettlebell even as it is within the air and get it to relaxation on the outside of your forearm.

2.Reverse the motion.

3.Repeat it 10 times.

Fine Tips:

1.Hold the kettlebell in unmarried hand, overhand function with thumb handling backwards.

2.Load the rear of the frame with the useful resource of using from the heels as you do the movement.

3.Engage your middle all through the motion. Squeeze your buttocks to straighten inside the final function, with out bending decrease once more.

4.Rotate the arm across the bell and not the opposite way round.

5. The bell moves up and down in a vertical route, near the body.

6. Engage the Latissimus dorsi muscle through way of way of squeezing the armpit at the top of the flow into.

7. Keep the movement easy and do now not bang the arm. In the final feature the elbow need to be in, wrist right now and kettlebell resting softly on the outside of your arm.

Kettlebell Floor to Shelf

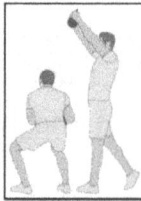

Effect: This exercise helps enhance entire-frame energy and movement in a multi-planar environment.

Difficulty Level: Beginner

Start Position: Hold the kettlebell with every hands underneath the cope with and keep it besides the hip. Squat on this function with ft hip width distance apart.

Steps:

1.Raise your body as you pivot and turn the torso inside the direction of the opposite aspect, elevating the kettlebell diagonally up, taking it above the alternative shoulder.

2.Pause on the top for a 2d.

3.Reverse the movement bringing kettlebell decrease again to the start function.

four.Repeat it 10 instances.

5.Repeat the gathering 10 instances at the opportunity aspect.

Fine Tips:

1.The motion must be gradual and controlled.

2.Keep your shoulders pulled decrease lower back and chest up within the path of the movement.

Overhead Squat

Effect: This exercising strengthens middle, hamstrings, quadriceps, glutes, shoulder and arm muscular tissues. It improves center balance.

Difficulty Level: Intermediate

Start Position: Stand tall with feet more than hip width distance apart and preserve kettlebell in right hand in overhead characteristic.

Steps:

1.Lower your frame into squat, preserving decrease again tall and kettlebell in overhead function.

2.Come decrease lower back to stand tall feature, pushing into the heels, retaining the kettlebell in overhead position.

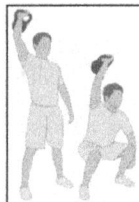

3.Return to the squat role.

4.Repeat it 10 instances.

5.Repeat 10 times on the left factor.

Fine Tips:

1.Keep your lower back tall and center engaged all through the movement.

2.The knees need to no longer bypass the ft beforehand inside the squat function.

three.Hold the kettlebell everyday in overhead characteristic inside the direction of the motion.

Double Kettlebell Squat with Press

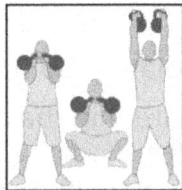

Effect: This exercise strengthens the middle, hamstrings, quadriceps, glutes, shoulders and arms muscle organizations. It improves middle balance and top and decrease limb mobility.

Difficulty Level: Intermediate

Start Position: Stand tall with toes extra than hip width distance apart. Hold kettlebells in every fingers in rack characteristic.

Steps:

1.Lower down your frame and get into a deep squat, pushing the hips again and down, Keeping kettlebells in rack role.

2.Push into the heels and are available to recognition function, maintaining kettlebells in rack function.

three.From the stand tall function, press the kettlebells immediately up in the direction of the ceiling, straightening the arms.

four.Lower the kettlebells to the rack feature, returning to the start characteristic.

5.Repeat the gathering 10 times.

Fine Tips:

1.Keep your decrease decrease again tall and middle engaged inside the route of the movement.

2.The knees want to not pass the ft beforehand within the squat characteristic.

Single Arm Kettlebell Snatch

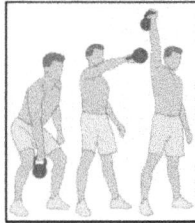

Effect: This exercise improves strength and balance of entire body. Strengthens shoulders and pinnacle again muscle corporations.

Difficulty Level: Intermediate

Start Position: Stand in a partial squat role together together together with your feet little wider than shoulder width aside. Hold the kettlebell inside the front of your frame, most of the legs, inside the overhand grip with arm immediately. Extend the alternative arm to the facet.

Steps:

1.Thrust your body up, coming to the status characteristic as you swing the kettlebell as a amazing deal because the shoulder stage. Turn your hand due to the fact the kettlebell reaches the shoulder degree and punch it up overhead. Catch the kettlebell in top function with arm immediately.

2.Pause at the top for a 2d.

3.Return to the begin feature.

4.Repeat the collection 10 times.

Fine Tips:

1.Control the kettle bell simply so it does no longer slam your arm at some level within the overhead movement.

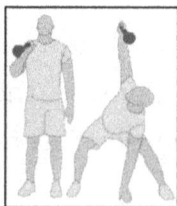

Kettlebell Windmill

Effect: It is a multi-planar exercising that strengthens the shoulder, triceps and trunk muscular tissues. It additionally improves power and stability of lower frame and center.

Difficulty Level: Intermediate

Start Position: Stand tall together along side your toes hip width distance aside. Hold the kettlebell inside the rack role.

Steps:

1.Step into a partial squat pushing the hips lower lower back and down, as you push the kettlebell overhead, straightening the arm, turning the kettlebell preserving palm in the course of the ceiling. Bring the possibility hand right down to stability the frame inside the front.

2.Pause at the pinnacle function.

3.Reverse the movement and go back to the begin function.

Fine Tips:

1.Do now not curve your again and reduce down at hips as to procure the ground.

Sumo Squat Swing

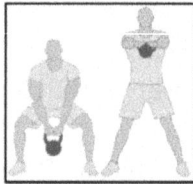

Effect: This workout strengthens the lower limbs, center and shoulder muscle organizations. It improves mobility of arms and decrease body. It improves middle stability.

Difficulty Level: Beginner

Start Position: Stand together together with your feet wider than hip width distance aside, ft pointing 20-30 tiers outwards. Hold the kettlebell in overhand grip in the front of your frame with hands instantly. Lower yourself in a partial squat.

Steps:

1.Thrust your hips in advance swinging the kettlebell ahead and upward to the shoulder degree. Return lower back to the squat function swinging the kettlebell down, within the identical motion.

2.Repeat this series 10 times.

Fine Tips:

1.Squatting is done thru pushing hips over again and down, not thru pushing knees ahead.

2.Keep your chest beforehand and center engaged at some stage within the motion.

three.The motion need to be initiated at hips, now not at knees.

four.Squeeze your glutes in pinnacle feature.

Kettlebell Bob and Weave

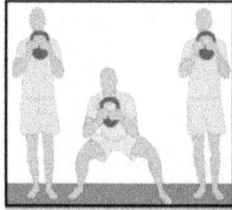

Effect: This workout strengthens the lateral hip and legs, hamstrings, quadriceps, back, trapezius, shoulder and center muscular tissues.

Difficulty Level: Intermediate

Start Position: Stand tall with ft hip width distance aside, retaining kettlebell at the chest degree with both hands.

Steps:

1.Keeping your returned tall and chest up, step to right factor lowering your hips down and decrease again. Hold the kettlebell constant on the chest role with shoulders down and over again.

2.Come returned to stand tall role as you are taking a few other step to proper thing.

three.Repeat the collection to the left issue.

4.Repeat the gathering 20 instances.

Fine Tips:

1.Keep your chest up, shoulders down and again and middle engaged at a few level in the motion.

2.Keep your frame weight on the heels and engage your hip muscle tissues as you do the movement.

3.The transition from popularity role to partial squat and again standing role ought to be gradual and managed.

4.Keep the kettlebell at the chest characteristic inside the path of the movement.

Deck Squat

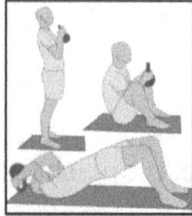

Effect: This is a complete body workout. It improves cardiovascular staying electricity. It strengthens the middle, shoulder, over again, glutes, hamstrings and quadriceps. It improves middle stability and hip mobility.

Difficulty Level: Advanced

Start Position: Stand tall with feet shoulder width aside and keep the kettlebell with every hands, near the chest.

Steps:

1.Lower yourself into the deep squat function, taking hips decrease again and down, maintaining the chest up and kettlebell near the chest.

2.Roll backwards preserving your heels firmly planted on the ground.

www.ingramcontent.com/pod-product-compliance
Lightning Source LLC
Chambersburg PA
CBHW062141020426
42335CB00013B/1293